Introduction

Finding Light in the Darkness: Understanding and Preventing Suicide, Self-Harm, and Coping with Bereavement

In our interconnected world, where the threads of human experience are woven together in complex and often challenging ways, the topics of suicide, self-harm, and bereavement remain profoundly significant and deeply personal. These issues touch lives in ways that are both visible and invisible, creating ripples of impact that extend through families, communities, and societies. This book, *Finding Light in the Darkness: Understanding and Preventing Suicide, Self-Harm, and Coping with Bereavement*, seeks to illuminate these dark corners with compassion, knowledge, and practical guidance.

Reflecting on the Importance of Discussing Suicide, Self-Harm, and Bereavement

The act of openly discussing suicide, self-harm, and bereavement is not only a necessary step towards understanding but also a powerful tool in breaking down the barriers of stigma and silence. It is through these conversations that we can begin to unravel the complexities of these issues, offering solace to those in pain and equipping communities with the tools they need to provide support. As someone deeply entrenched in the fields of coaching and counselling, I have witnessed first-hand the transformative power that comes from addressing these subjects with honesty and empathy.

In Ireland and the UK, where mental health awareness is growing yet still faces significant challenges, there is an urgent need for resources that bridge the gap between knowledge and action. This book aims to be that bridge, providing insights, strategies, and support for individuals and their loved ones navigating these difficult journeys.

Setting the Tone for a Compassionate and Informative Exploration

Our exploration begins with an understanding that each person's experience is unique. The pain and suffering that accompany suicidal thoughts, self-harming behaviours, and the grief of losing a loved one to suicide are deeply personal and multifaceted. This book is designed to offer a compassionate and comprehensive exploration of these topics.

Drawing on my extensive background in coaching, counselling, and mental health advocacy, this book weaves together theoretical knowledge with practical applications. The goal is not only to inform but also to inspire hope and resilience. By addressing these issues head-on, we aim to empower readers to take proactive steps towards prevention, intervention, and healing.

A Compassionate Approach to Difficult Topics

This book is structured to guide readers through a journey of understanding and support. We begin by examining the prevalence and risk factors of suicide, dispelling myths, and providing a clear picture of the realities faced by those at risk. We then look into the behaviours and motivations behind self-harm, offering strategies for Recognising and addressing these actions.

The impact of suicide on loved ones is profound, and this book explores the unique challenges of bereavement after suicide, offering coping strategies and support mechanisms. We also provide practical guidance for those supporting individuals affected by suicide, emphasizing the importance of empathy and non-judgmental support.

In the later chapters, we focus on prevention strategies and early intervention, highlighting the importance of community outreach and mental health education. Addressing the stigma associated with mental health issues is a recurring theme, as we advocate for a more understanding and supportive society.

Conclusion

Finding Light in the Darkness is more than just a book; it is a call to action. It is an invitation to join a conversation that has the potential to save lives and foster healing. Through the pages of this book, we seek to provide a beacon of hope, guiding readers towards understanding, prevention, and recovery.

In writing this book, I draw upon my personal and professional experiences to offer a resource that is both informative and compassionate. It is my hope that this book will serve as a valuable tool for individuals, families, and communities, helping them to navigate the complexities of suicide, self-harm, and bereavement with empathy and resilience.

About the Author

Seán O'Connor is a highly skilled and seasoned professional in the field of coaching and counselling. With many years of experience, Seán has made a significant impact on the lives of numerous individuals, guiding them towards personal growth, emotional well-being, and transformative change.

Seán is the owner of Seán O'Connor Coaching, a coaching practice specializing in empowering individuals to reach their full potential. With a passion for personal and professional development, Seán has been dedicating himself to the field of coaching for the past six years.

Since September 2017, Seán has been actively involved in coaching, partnering with clients in a thought-provoking and creative process. Through this collaborative approach, he inspires individuals to unlock their untapped sources of imagination, productivity, and leadership. Seán firmly believes in the transformative power of coaching and its ability to help individuals maximize their personal and professional capabilities.

In addition to his coaching practice, Seán also conducts training workshops and seminars in various areas. These include resilience and stress management, time management and personal effectiveness, as well as communication and interview skills. Seán's expertise in these areas allows him to provide valuable insights and practical strategies to individuals and organisations seeking to enhance their performance.

With a deep understanding of human resources, Seán also holds a role as a Coach with the HSE, further validating his expertise and credibility in the field. His holistic approach to coaching encompasses a range of areas, enabling him to guide clients through both personal and professional challenges.

Also, as a humanistic-trained counsellor he focuses on the individual's inherent capacity for growth and self-actualization. This approach emphasises the importance of the therapeutic relationship and utilizes techniques such as empathy, genuineness, and unconditional positive regard to create a safe and supportive space for clients to explore their thoughts, feelings, and experiences.

During his time as a Counsellor at HMP Forest Bank, he navigated the challenging environment of a Category B prison in the UK. In this capacity, he provided counselling sessions to adult offenders grappling with complex needs, encompassing issues related to mental health, addiction, depression, self-harm, and suicidal ideation.

Subsequently, in his role as a Counsellor at Acorn Counselling he undertook similar responsibilities within a small voluntary organisation based in Manchester. At Acorn Counselling, he engaged actively with individuals, conducted complex therapeutic assessments, built trust with clients, and provided counselling sessions. His role also encompassed referring clients to healthcare professionals, ongoing monitoring of clients' responses to counselling with meticulous maintenance of clinical records.

His deep understanding of human psychology and emotional dynamics allows him to create a trusting therapeutic alliance, where clients feel heard, validated, and supported throughout their healing journey.

Seán has successfully guided clients through trauma, grief, anxiety, depression, and other mental health challenges, equipping them with tools and coping strategies to regain their well-being and live fulfilling lives.

Seán is known for their warmth, professionalism, and genuine passion for helping others. His ability to create a nurturing and empowering therapeutic environment allows clients to feel supported, validated, and inspired to embark on a transformative journey of self-discovery and growth.

In conclusion, Seán is a highly respected and experienced coach and counsellor, equipped with the wisdom, skills, and compassion to guide individuals towards personal transformation, emotional well-being, and empowered living.

Career background

Seán O'Connor is a highly accomplished health professional with a diverse range of experiences and a strong commitment to making a positive impact in the field of health and well-being. Currently serving as a Project Manager in Arts & Health within the Health Service Executive (HSE), Seán is dedicated to exploring the intersections between creativity and health to enhance the well-being of individuals and staff.

In addition to his role in Arts & Health, Seán holds a significant position as a lay member on tribunal panels for the Mental Health Commission. This involvement allows him to contribute to the fair and just assessment of mental health cases, ensuring that the rights and well-being of individuals are protected.

Seán is also deeply passionate about road safety and has developed the Drive Aware Programme (DAP) as a means to effect positive changes in attitudes and behaviours related to impaired, dangerous, and careless driving. Through his program, Seán aims to promote responsible driving practices and reduce the risks associated with reckless behaviour on the roads. His dedication to enhancing road safety has led him to deliver the Drive Aware Programme throughout the country.

As the founder of Seán O'Connor Coaching, Seán offers personalized one-on-one coaching sessions and conducts training workshops and seminars. Leveraging his extensive knowledge and experience, he empowers individuals to overcome challenges, improve their well-being, and achieve personal and professional growth.

Throughout his career, Seán has held various impactful positions. He served as a Project Manager with the HSE National Clinical Programme for People with Disability, where he played a pivotal role in improving healthcare services and support for individuals with disabilities.

As a Task Force Manager in the HSE Drugs & Alcohol sector, Seán contributed to the development and implementation of strategies to address substance abuse issues within the community.

His previous roles also include serving as the Director of the Dyslexia Association of Ireland, where he championed the rights and needs of individuals with dyslexia, and as the Chairperson and Director of Pieta House, an organisation dedicated to preventing suicide and providing support to those in crisis.

Furthermore,

Seán has a unique background in the legal field, having served as a sitting Magistrate/Justice of the Peace within Her Majesty's Court Service. He brings a profound understanding of the criminal justice system and leverages this knowledge to make fair and informed decisions.

Seán's expertise extends to the field of addiction counselling, having worked as an Addiction Counsellor in both community and prison settings. He has provided vital support and guidance to individuals struggling with addiction, helping them on their journey towards recovery. Seán has also contributed to the provision of counselling services within the prison setting, recognising the importance of addressing mental health needs in such environments.

Additionally, Seán has made valuable contributions to the criminal justice system as a Drug & Alcohol worker with Probation Services. His work in this capacity focused on assisting individuals in overcoming addiction, reintegrating into society, and reducing reoffending rates.

Media work within TV and radio has provided Seán with a platform to raise awareness about various health and social issues. He has utilized these mediums to educate and inform the public, advocating for positive change and promoting well-being.

Seán's career began in engineering, where he embarked on a four-year apprenticeship as a fresh-faced sixteen-year-old. He gained invaluable experience working for a large multinational Oil and Gas company, further developing his skills and contributing to the industry.

With an impressive array of experiences spanning healthcare, project management, coaching, counselling, advocacy, and engineering, Seán O'Connor embodies a passionate and dedicated health professional committed to improving the lives of individuals and communities. His multifaceted background and expertise enable him to address complex challenges, inspire positive change, and empower others to reach their full potential.

And for further insights into Sean's career to date please visit LinkedIn

https://www.linkedin.com/in/sean-oconnor/

Here's a quick rundown of Seán's publications to date:

A Therapist's Guide to a Little Bit of Everything: Is a comprehensive and invaluable resource designed to support therapists in navigating a wide range of topics and issues they may encounter in their practice.

From Struggle to Strength: Resilience is a quality deeply ingrained in the human spirit. It is the remarkable ability to withstand adversity, recover from setbacks, and emerge stronger than before. In this book, we embark on a journey to understand the essence of resilience, its significance, and the profound impact it can have on our lives

Feck Off Anxiety: As someone deeply invested in the fields of Coaching and Counselling, I have witnessed first-hand the profound impact that anxiety can have on individuals, families, and communities.

Feck Off Overthinking: Looks into the intricate web of overthinking, seeking not only to comprehend its depths but to provide you, the reader.

Feck Off Depression: This book looks into the complex landscape of depression, unravelling its many facets and providing insights into its various forms, from major depressive disorder and persistent depressive disorder to the cyclical highs and lows of bipolar disorder.

Feck Off Stress: A guide that doesn't just help you cope with stress but empowers you to conquer it.

Leading in Healthcare Management and Leadership in the UK and Ireland: Exploring the intricacies of healthcare leadership and management, shedding light on effective practices in this ever-evolving field.

Leading with Purpose: A Guide to Being an Effective Chairperson in the Charity Sector of the UK and Ireland - Offering guidance to aspiring and current chairpersons, emphasizing the importance of purpose-driven leadership in the non-profit sector.

Empowering Voices: A Comprehensive Guide to Becoming a Freelance Contributor in Drug and Alcohol Addiction Journalism a resource for aspiring freelance journalists interested in covering the crucial topics of drug and alcohol addiction.

Breaking the Chains: A Comprehensive Guide to Addiction Counselling in Ireland and the UK - Shedding light on effective counselling techniques and strategies to support individuals in overcoming addiction.

Shattering Stigma: This book aims to provide a comprehensive section of mental health services in Ireland, looking into the intricacies of assessment, diagnosis, and treatment.

Drive Aware: "Safer roads for a safer society" - This has been the driving principle behind the ambitious initiative known as the Drive Aware program in Ireland.

Empowering Change: A Project Manager's Perspective on the Disability Sector in Ireland: This comprehensive induction provides you with a strong foundation to navigate your role as a Project Manager in the disability sector.

Balancing Justice: A Magistrate's Journey - Sharing my personal experiences and insights as a magistrate, highlighting the challenges and rewards of serving in the legal system.

Mastering Life Coaching: A Comprehensive Guide for Professional Coaches - Equipping life coaches with the necessary tools and knowledge to empower their clients and facilitate positive change.

Clearing the Air: Smoking Cessation Services in the UK and their Benefits to Society - Advocating for the importance of smoking cessation and exploring the valuable services available to individuals looking to quit smoking.

My Journey with Ulcerative Colitis: From Fear to Understanding: Seán navigates the ups and downs of life with ulcerative colitis – exploring the physical, emotional, and practical aspects of managing this condition with grace and resilience.

Embracing Dyslexia: Building Strengths, Overcoming Challenges: The book begins by defining dyslexia as a specific learning difference that affects reading, writing, and information processing, emphasizing that it is not indicative of intelligence but rather a neurological difference in language processing.

Engineering Excellence: Unveiling the Potential of the Gas and Petroleum Industry' - An exploration of the gas and petroleum industry, revealing the incredible potential and advancements within this vital sector.

All of the above publications can be found at

https://www.amazon.co.uk/~/e/B0C8G4ZN94

Where you can contact him

Seán O'Connor Coaching

https://www.seanoconnorcoaching.com/

Drive Aware Ireland

https://www.driveaware.ie/

Chapter Outline:

1. **Introduction – Page 16**

Reflecting on the importance of discussing suicide, self-harm, and bereavement.

Setting the tone for a compassionate and informative exploration of these interconnected topics.

2. **Understanding Suicide – Page 20**

Statistics and prevalence of suicide globally and within specific populations.

Discussion of risk factors, warning signs, and contributing mental health factors.

Myths and misconceptions about suicide.

3. **Self-Harm: Understanding the Behaviour – Page 29**

Defining self-harm and exploring its relationship with mental health.

Motivations behind self-harm and common methods.

The link between self-harm and suicide risk.

4. **Recognising Self-Harm and Suicide Risk – Page 36**

Identifying signs of self-harm and suicidal ideation in oneself and others.

When and how to seek help for individuals struggling with self-harm or suicidal thoughts.

1. Reflecting on the Importance of Discussing Suicide, Self-Harm, and Bereavement

In the realm of mental health, certain topics evoke discomfort and silence. Suicide, self-harm, and the aftermath of bereavement are among these subjects, often veiled in stigma and misconceptions. Yet, the imperative to openly and compassionately discuss these issues cannot be overstated. It is within these conversations that lives can be saved, suffering alleviated, and healing fostered.

The urgency of addressing suicide, self-harm, and bereavement arises from their profound impact on individuals, families, and communities. Suicide remains a leading cause of death worldwide, with devastating consequences that extend far beyond the individual act. Each life lost to suicide represents a unique narrative of pain, despair, and unfulfilled potential. By shining a light on suicide, we acknowledge its prevalence and dispel the myth that it is a taboo or shameful topic.

Self-harm, often a precursor to suicidal behaviour, is another facet of mental distress that demands our attention. Despite its prevalence, self-harm is frequently misunderstood and marginalised. Understanding the motivations behind self-harm, such as emotional regulation or coping with overwhelming feelings, is crucial for effective intervention and support.

Equally significant is the profound impact of suicide on those left behind—the bereaved who grapple with unimaginable grief, guilt, and unanswered questions. Bereavement after suicide carries its own set of challenges, including stigma and societal judgment. Open dialogue about suicide bereavement is essential for fostering empathy and offering meaningful support to those affected.

As a society, we must confront the uncomfortable truths surrounding suicide, self-harm, and bereavement with empathy and courage. Silence perpetuates stigma and hinders prevention efforts. By engaging in open, informed conversations, we create opportunities for education, empathy, and intervention.

Discussing suicide, self-harm, and bereavement is not just about acknowledging the pain; it is about taking proactive steps towards prevention and healing. It is about recognising that mental health challenges are part of the human experience and deserve compassionate, non-judgmental responses.

For those struggling with suicidal thoughts or self-harm, open dialogue can be life-saving. It offers a lifeline a reminder that help is available and that one is not alone in their struggles. For the bereaved, discussion fosters validation of their grief and reduces feelings of isolation.

Ultimately, discussing suicide, self-harm, and bereavement is an act of compassion a declaration that every individual's life is precious and worthy of support. It is a call to action to dismantle stigma, promote mental health literacy, and cultivate resilience.

In this book, we embark on a journey of understanding and prevention a journey guided by empathy, evidence based strategies, and narratives of hope.

Setting the Tone: A Compassionate and Informative Exploration

In embarking on an exploration of suicide, self-harm, and bereavement, we are guided by a commitment to compassion, empathy, and understanding. These interconnected topics demand more than academic scrutiny; they require a heartfelt engagement that acknowledges the depth of human suffering and the potential for healing and resilience.

The tone of our exploration is one of deep empathy an acknowledgment of the complexities and challenges inherent in mental health struggles. We approach these sensitive topics not with judgment or sensationalism but with a genuine desire to foster awareness, offer support, and ultimately prevent unnecessary loss of life.

Compassion forms the cornerstone of our discussion. We recognise that behind every statistic lies a unique individual with a story shaped by pain, vulnerability, and, ultimately, a quest for hope. By approaching these topics with compassion, we honour the lived experiences of those affected and convey a message of solidarity and understanding.

Our exploration is also informed by a commitment to providing accurate, evidence-based information. We seek to dispel myths and misconceptions surrounding suicide and self-harm, replacing ignorance with knowledge and fear with empathy. Through informed discussion, we empower individuals to recognise warning signs, initiate conversations, and access appropriate resources.

Amidst the gravity of these topics, we emphasise the importance of fostering hope and resilience. While acknowledging the profound challenges of mental health struggles.

Furthermore, our exploration is intended to catalyse action. By discussing these topics openly and honestly, we aim to mobilise individuals, families, and communities to prioritise mental health and advocate for improved support systems. Prevention and intervention are not passive endeavours; they require proactive engagement and collective commitment.

As we navigate this terrain together, let us hold space for vulnerability and authenticity. Let us listen with open hearts, speak with empathy, and act with purpose. Together, we can challenge stigma, promote understanding, and cultivate a culture of compassion that values mental health and well-being.

In the pages that follow, we invite you to join us on a journey of discovery one that embraces complexity, confronts stigma, and celebrates the resilience of the human spirit. Through compassionate dialogue and informed action, we can find light in the darkness and foster a future where every individual feels seen, supported, and valued.

2. Understanding Suicide: Statistics and Prevalence

Suicide is a profound public health issue that manifests differently across regions and populations. Examining the statistics and prevalence of suicide provides critical insights into its impact on communities and informs targeted prevention strategies.

Global Overview:

Globally, suicide accounts for approximately 800,000 deaths annually, making it a significant contributor to mortality. The World Health Organisation (WHO) estimates that suicide rates vary widely by country, with high-income nations generally reporting higher rates than low- and middle-income countries. However, suicide is a complex phenomenon influenced by social, economic, and cultural factors.

Ireland and the UK:

Ireland: In Ireland, suicide rates have been a concern in recent years, particularly among certain demographic groups. According to the Central Statistics Office (CSO), Ireland's suicide rate was 10.1 per 100,000 population in 2020, with a higher rate among males than females. The age group most affected by suicide in Ireland is young adults aged 15-34, although suicide rates are also significant among older age groups.

Factors contributing to suicide risk in Ireland include social isolation, economic hardship, substance abuse, and mental health challenges. Efforts to address suicide prevention in Ireland have included increased mental health awareness campaigns, community-based support services, and initiatives targeting high-risk populations.

United Kingdom (UK): In the UK, suicide rates also exhibit variations by region and demographic characteristics. According to the Office for National Statistics (ONS), the UK's suicide rate was 11.0 per 100,000 population in 2020, with higher rates among males than females. The highest suicide rates are observed in middle-aged men, although suicide affects individuals across the lifespan.

Age-specific trends highlight the vulnerability of certain age groups to suicide. In both Ireland and the UK, young adults aged 15-34 and middle-aged adults face elevated suicide risk, often attributed to factors such as economic uncertainty, relationship difficulties, and mental health disorders.

Other Information:

Gender Disparities: Across both Ireland and the UK, males consistently account for a higher proportion of suicide deaths compared to females. This gender disparity underscores the importance of addressing societal expectations related to masculinity and help-seeking behaviours.

Mental Health Factors: Mental health disorders, such as depression, anxiety, and substance abuse, are significant risk factors for suicide in both countries. Improving access to mental health services and reducing stigma surrounding mental illness are critical components of suicide prevention efforts.

Community Interventions: Suicide prevention initiatives in Ireland and the UK emphasise community-based interventions, peer support networks, and early intervention strategies targeting high-risk individuals and populations.

Understanding the nuanced landscape of suicide within specific populations is essential for designing effective prevention programs and support services.

By addressing underlying risk factors and promoting mental health resilience, we can work towards reducing suicide rates and fostering supportive communities.

In the subsequent chapters, we will look deeper into risk factors, warning signs, and evidence-based interventions aimed at preventing suicide and promoting mental well-being across Ireland, the UK, and beyond.

Discussion of Risk Factors, Warning Signs, and Contributing Mental Health Factors

Suicide is a complex and multifaceted phenomenon influenced by a combination of individual, social, and psychological factors. Understanding the interplay of risk factors and warning signs is crucial for identifying individuals at heightened risk and implementing targeted intervention strategies.

Risk Factors:

Mental Health Disorders: Mental illnesses such as depression, bipolar disorder, schizophrenia, and substance use disorders significantly increase the risk of suicide. These disorders can impair coping mechanisms, distort perceptions of reality, and lead to feelings of hopelessness and despair.

Previous Suicide Attempts: Individuals with a history of suicide attempts are at increased risk of future suicidal behaviour. Previous suicide attempts are among the strongest predictors of completed suicide.

Family History of Suicide: A family history of suicide or suicidal behaviour may contribute to an individual's susceptibility to suicidal thoughts and behaviours due to genetic, environmental, or learned factors.

Chronic Illness or Pain: Chronic physical illnesses, disabilities, or persistent pain conditions can contribute to feelings of despair and hopelessness, increasing the risk of suicide.

Social Isolation: Lack of social support, loneliness, or perceived social rejection can exacerbate feelings of worthlessness and contribute to suicidal ideation.

Trauma and Adverse Life Events: Experiencing trauma, abuse, loss of a loved one, or significant life stressors can overwhelm coping mechanisms and increase vulnerability to suicidal thoughts.

Access to Lethal Means: Easy access to firearms, medications, or other lethal methods increases the risk of impulsive suicide attempts.

Substance Abuse: Alcohol and drug misuse can impair judgment, exacerbate underlying mental health issues, and increase impulsivity, elevating the risk of suicidal behaviour.

Warning Signs:

Expressing Suicidal Ideation: Verbalising thoughts of suicide, even indirectly, should always be taken seriously and viewed as a clear warning sign.

Behavioural Changes: Sudden changes in behaviour, mood, or personality, such as increased withdrawal, recklessness, or giving away possessions, may indicate distress.

Isolation and Withdrawal: Social withdrawal, avoidance of usual activities, or disengagement from relationships may signal underlying emotional turmoil.

Hopelessness and Despair: Expressions of hopelessness about the future, feeling trapped, or believing that life is not worth living are significant warning signs.

Sleep Disturbances: Insomnia, hypersomnia, or significant changes in sleep patterns can be indicators of emotional distress.

Self-Harm: Engagement in self-harming behaviours, such as cutting or burning, may be a precursor to suicidal behaviour and should not be dismissed.

Increased Substance Use: Escalating alcohol or drug use may indicate attempts to cope with emotional pain.

Contributing Mental Health Factors:

Depression and Mood Disorders: Persistent feelings of sadness, worthlessness, and loss of interest in activities are hallmark features of depression and major risk factors for suicide.

Anxiety Disorders: Chronic anxiety, panic attacks, and obsessive-compulsive behaviours can contribute to suicidal thoughts and behaviours, especially in the context of overwhelming distress.

Personality Disorders: Certain personality traits, such as impulsivity, emotional instability, and interpersonal difficulties, may increase vulnerability to suicidal behaviour.

Psychotic Disorders: Psychotic symptoms, including hallucinations or delusions, can lead to distorted perceptions of reality and increase suicide risk.

Substance Use Disorders: Co-occurring substance abuse and mental health disorders significantly elevate suicide risk due to impaired judgment and increased impulsivity.

Understanding the intricate web of risk factors, warning signs, and underlying mental health factors associated with suicide is essential for effective prevention and intervention efforts. By promoting awareness, destigmatising mental health discussions, and fostering supportive environments, we can work towards reducing the incidence of suicide and saving lives.

In the subsequent chapters, we will look into evidence-based strategies for suicide prevention, crisis intervention, and promoting mental well-being across diverse populations.

Myths and Misconceptions about Suicide

Suicide is a deeply complex and sensitive topic often shrouded in myths and misconceptions. Addressing these myths is essential for promoting understanding, reducing stigma, and fostering effective suicide prevention strategies.

Myth #1: "People who talk about suicide are not serious and won't actually do it."

Fact: Verbalising thoughts of suicide should always be taken seriously. Many individuals who die by suicide have communicated their intentions or distress beforehand. It is crucial to listen non-judgmentally and offer support to those expressing suicidal ideation.

Myth #2: "Suicide only affects individuals with mental health disorders."

Fact: While mental health disorders are significant risk factors for suicide, suicide can affect anyone regardless of their mental health status. External stressors, traumatic life events, and acute crises can also contribute to suicidal thoughts and behaviours.

Myth #3: "People who attempt suicide are selfish or seeking attention."

Fact: Suicide is often a desperate attempt to escape overwhelming emotional pain and distress. Individuals contemplating suicide may feel hopeless, trapped, and unable to see alternative solutions. It is not a selfish act but a manifestation of deep suffering.

Myth #4: "Once someone is suicidal, there's nothing you can do to help."

Fact: Intervention and support can make a profound difference in preventing suicide. Providing empathetic listening, connecting individuals to professional help, and ensuring access to mental health resources can save lives.

Myth #5: "Talking about suicide will plant the idea in someone's mind."

Fact: Openly discussing suicide in a supportive and non-judgmental manner can actually reduce stigma and encourage help-seeking behaviours. Ignoring or avoiding the topic may perpetuate feelings of isolation and shame.

Myth #6: "Suicide rates are highest during the winter holidays."

Fact: While holiday stressors can exacerbate emotional distress, suicide rates tend to peak in the spring and early summer months. It is essential to provide support and resources year-round, not just during the holiday season.

Myth #7: "Once someone decides to die by suicide, there's no way to stop them."

Fact: Suicide is preventable. Most individuals experiencing suicidal thoughts are ambivalent about ending their lives and may be open to receiving help. Early intervention and support can offer hope and alternatives to suicide.

Myth #8: "Only certain types of people die by suicide."

Fact: Suicide affects individuals of all ages, genders, ethnicities, and socio-economic backgrounds. No one is immune to the risk of suicide, and everyone deserves compassion and support.

Myth #9: "Suicide is an impulsive act."

Fact: While impulsivity can contribute to some suicide attempts, most suicidal behaviours are preceded by underlying mental health issues, distress, and coping challenges. Suicide is often a complex process involving a combination of factors.

Myth #10: "Suicide is a normal response to stress or hardship."

Fact: Suicide is not a normal or inevitable response to adversity. It is a tragic outcome of untreated mental health disorders, overwhelming distress, and unmet psychological needs.

Challenging these myths and misconceptions is critical for promoting an accurate understanding of suicide and fostering compassionate responses to individuals in crisis. By debunking stigma and increasing awareness, we can create supportive communities that prioritise mental health and well-being.

In the subsequent chapters, we will continue to address common misconceptions and provide evidence-based strategies for suicide prevention and intervention.

3. Self-Harm: Understanding the Behaviour

Self-harm, also known as self-injury or self-mutilation, refers to intentional, non-suicidal acts of harming one's body, often as a way to cope with emotional distress or overwhelming feelings. Understanding the nature of self-harm is essential for identifying underlying issues and providing appropriate support and intervention.

Defining Self-Harm:

Self-harm encompasses a range of behaviours in which individuals deliberately inflict injury or damage to their bodies without the intent to die. Common forms of self-harm include cutting, burning, hitting, scratching, and picking at skin. Self-harm may be hidden or discreet, and individuals often go to great lengths to conceal their injuries.

Self-harm is not a suicidal act, although it can co-occur with suicidal thoughts or intentions. It is primarily a maladaptive coping mechanism used to regulate emotions, alleviate psychological distress, or gain a sense of control over overwhelming feelings. Individuals engaging in self-harm may report temporary relief or distraction from emotional pain following the behaviour.

Exploring its Relationship with Mental Health:

Self-harm is strongly associated with underlying mental health issues, particularly mood disorders, anxiety disorders, and trauma-related disorders. Common mental health conditions linked to self-harm include:

Depression: Persistent feelings of sadness, hopelessness, and worthlessness may drive individuals to self-harm as a means of coping with emotional pain.

Borderline Personality Disorder (BPD): Individuals with BPD often use self-harm as a way to regulate intense emotions and alleviate feelings of emptiness or instability.

Post-Traumatic Stress Disorder (PTSD): Trauma survivors may engage in self-harm as a maladaptive coping strategy to manage distressing memories and intrusive thoughts.

Eating Disorders: Self-harm behaviours, such as cutting or burning, may co-occur with eating disorders as a method of exerting control or managing body image concerns.

Anxiety Disorders: Individuals experiencing chronic anxiety or panic attacks may resort to self-harm as a temporary relief from overwhelming fear and tension.

Self-harm serves as a coping mechanism to express and manage intense emotions that feel unmanageable or intolerable. It can also serve as a way to communicate distress when verbal expression is challenging or inadequate.

It is important to note that self-harm is a symptom of underlying distress and should not be dismissed or minimised. Addressing the root causes of self-harm requires a comprehensive approach that includes therapeutic interventions, emotional support, and skill-building to develop healthier coping strategies.

By understanding the complex relationship between self-harm and mental health, we can better support individuals struggling with these behaviours and promote effective pathways to recovery and healing.

In the subsequent chapters, we will look into deeper into the assessment, management, and treatment of self-harm behaviours, emphasizing the importance of compassionate care and holistic interventions.

Motivations behind Self-Harm and Common Methods

Self-harm is a complex behaviour driven by various motivations, emotions, and underlying psychological factors. Understanding the motivations behind self-harm is essential for developing effective interventions and providing compassionate support to individuals struggling with these behaviours.

Motivations Behind Self-Harm:

Emotional Regulation: One of the primary motivations behind self-harm is the desire to regulate intense emotions or alleviate emotional distress. Individuals may use self-harm as a coping mechanism to cope with overwhelming feelings of sadness, anxiety, anger, or numbness.

Coping with Trauma: Self-harm can be a maladaptive response to past trauma or abuse. Individuals may use self-injury as a way to manage intrusive memories, flashbacks, or dissociative experiences associated with trauma.

Communication of Distress: For some individuals, self-harm serves as a non-verbal way to communicate emotional pain or distress that feels difficult to express verbally. It may be a way to seek attention or convey internal struggles to others.

Sense of Control: Engaging in self-harm may provide a temporary sense of control over overwhelming emotions or life circumstances. It can serve as a way to exert agency in situations perceived as chaotic or uncontrollable.

Self-Punishment: Feelings of guilt, shame, or self-loathing may lead individuals to self-harm as a form of self-punishment or self-sabotage. It may be linked to negative self-perceptions or distorted beliefs about deserving pain.

Release of Endorphins: Physical pain caused by self-harm can trigger the release of endorphins, which temporarily alleviate emotional pain and create a sense of relief or euphoria.

Distraction from Psychological Pain: Some individuals use self-harm as a distraction from overwhelming psychological pain or intrusive thoughts. The act of self-injury may provide a brief reprieve from internal turmoil.

Common Methods of Self-Harm:

Cutting: Using sharp objects (such as razor blades, knives, or scissors) to make cuts or incisions on the skin, typically on arms, legs, or other accessible body parts.

Burning: Applying heat or flame (e.g., with lighters, matches, or heated objects) to the skin to cause burns and tissue damage.

Hitting or Banging: Striking oneself against hard surfaces or objects to induce physical pain and bruising.

Scratching or Picking: Using fingernails or sharp objects to scratch or pick at the skin, resulting in wounds or abrasions.

Hair Pulling (Trichotillomania): Pulling out hair from the scalp, eyebrows, or other body parts as a compulsive behaviour.

Biting: Biting oneself or objects to cause pain and injury.

Ingesting Harmful Substances: Ingesting toxic substances or medications in an act of self-harm.

It's important to recognise that self-harm is not limited to these methods and can manifest in various forms based on individual preferences and accessibility of tools. Each act of self-harm is a unique expression of distress and requires individualised assessment and intervention.

By understanding the motivations behind self-harm and recognising common methods, caregivers, mental health professionals, and support networks can provide empathetic support, address underlying issues, and facilitate pathways to healthier coping strategies and emotional regulation.

In the subsequent chapters, we will explore evidence-based approaches for assessing and addressing self-harm behaviours, emphasising the importance of trauma-informed care, therapeutic interventions, and building resilience.

The Link Between Self-Harm and Suicide Risk

Self-harm and suicide are interconnected behaviours that share complex underlying factors and psychological distress. Understanding the relationship between self-harm and suicide risk is essential for effective assessment, intervention, and prevention strategies.

Nature of the Link:

Gateway to Suicide: While self-harm is not inherently suicidal, individuals who engage in self-harm are at an increased risk of suicidal thoughts and behaviours. Self-harm can serve as a precursor or warning sign of escalating distress and unmet mental health needs.

Coping Mechanism: Both self-harm and suicide can be maladaptive coping mechanisms used to manage overwhelming emotions and psychological pain. Individuals may initially use self-harm to regulate emotions but may escalate to suicidal thoughts if underlying issues remain unaddressed.

Underlying Mental Health Disorders: Self-harm and suicide are often associated with common mental health disorders, such as depression, anxiety, borderline personality disorder (BPD), and post-traumatic stress disorder (PTSD). These disorders contribute to increased vulnerability and distress.

Interpersonal Factors: Relationship difficulties, social isolation, bullying, and interpersonal conflicts can exacerbate feelings of despair and hopelessness, increasing the risk of both self-harm and suicide.

Suicide Risk Factors Associated with Self-Harm:

History of Self-Harm: Individuals with a history of self-harm are at a significantly higher risk of suicidal behaviour, especially if self-harm escalates in severity or frequency over time.

Severity of Self-Harm: The severity and lethality of self-harm methods (e.g., deep cutting, burning) may indicate heightened suicide risk, as individuals may inadvertently cause serious harm or death.

Underlying Mental Health Disorders: Co-occurring mental health disorders, particularly mood disorders and personality disorders, increase suicide risk among individuals engaging in self-harm.

Isolation and Lack of Social Support: Feelings of social isolation, perceived burdensomeness, and lack of supportive relationships contribute to increased suicide risk.

Access to Means: Easy access to lethal means (e.g., firearms, medications) increases the likelihood of suicide attempts among individuals experiencing distress.

Assessment and Intervention:

Effective assessment and intervention for individuals engaging in self-harm should include thorough evaluation of suicide risk factors and mental health needs. Mental health professionals should:

Conduct comprehensive risk assessments to identify underlying psychological factors and suicidal ideation.

Establish safety plans and crisis interventions tailored to individual needs and risk levels.

Provide evidence-based therapies, such as dialectical behaviour therapy (DBT), cognitive-behavioural therapy (CBT), and trauma-focused interventions, to address underlying issues and promote healthier coping strategies.

Foster supportive environments and strengthen social connections to reduce isolation and promote resilience.

Collaborate with multidisciplinary teams to ensure holistic care and ongoing support.

By recognising the link between self-harm and suicide risk and addressing underlying vulnerabilities, we can enhance suicide prevention efforts and promote mental health resilience among at-risk populations.

In the subsequent chapters, we will explore practical strategies for assessing, managing, and preventing suicide risk among individuals struggling with self-harm behaviours, emphasizing the importance of compassionate care and proactive intervention.

4. Recognising Self-Harm and Suicide Risk: Identifying Signs

Recognising signs of self-harm and suicidal ideation is crucial for early intervention and providing support to individuals in distress. Awareness of warning signs empowers individuals, caregivers, and communities to take proactive steps towards suicide prevention and mental health promotion.

Identifying Signs of Self-Harm:

Physical Signs:

Unexplained cuts, bruises, or burns, particularly in discrete areas of the body.

Wearing clothing that conceals body parts (e.g., long sleeves, pants) regardless of weather.

Frequent bandaging or hiding injuries without a plausible explanation.

Behavioural Signs:

Withdrawal from social activities or isolating oneself from family and friends.

Sudden changes in mood, such as increased irritability, agitation, or emotional volatility.

Engaging in secretive behaviours or spending excessive time alone in isolation.

Emotional Signs:

Expressions of hopelessness, worthlessness, or self-loathing.

Difficulty coping with stress or experiencing overwhelming emotions.

Verbal hints or statements suggesting self-harm as a coping mechanism.

Psychological Signs:

Increased use of alcohol or drugs as a means of coping with emotional distress.

Compulsive behaviours, such as hair-pulling (trichotillomania) or skin-picking (dermatillomania), indicative of underlying distress.

Identifying Signs of Suicidal Ideation:

Verbal Cues:

Direct statements about wanting to die or end one's life (e.g., "I wish I weren't here anymore," "I want to disappear").

Expressions of hopelessness or believing that life has no purpose or meaning.

Behavioural Changes:

Giving away personal belongings or making arrangements as if preparing for departure.

Reckless behaviour or engaging in dangerous activities without regard for personal safety.

Emotional Indicators:

Sudden shifts in mood, including extreme sadness, despair, or emotional numbness.

Expressions of feeling trapped or overwhelmed by life circumstances.

Withdrawal and Isolation:

Avoidance of social interactions and reluctance to engage in usual activities.

Spending prolonged periods alone or exhibiting signs of social detachment.

Recognising Signs in Oneself:

Acknowledge and validate feelings of distress or emotional pain.

Be honest and open about thoughts of self-harm or suicide with trusted individuals.

Seek professional help from mental health providers or crisis support services.

Recognising Signs in Others:

Approach the individual with empathy and non-judgmental support.

Listen actively and validate their feelings without minimizing or dismissing their experiences.

Encourage seeking help from mental health professionals or crisis intervention services.

Responding to Signs of Self-Harm and Suicide Risk:

Express concern and offer support in a non-confrontational manner.

Encourage open communication and prioritise safety by removing access to means of self-harm.

Connect the individual with professional resources, such as crisis hotlines, therapists, or support groups.

By recognising early warning signs of self-harm and suicidal ideation, we can intervene effectively, provide compassionate support, and ultimately save lives. It is essential to prioritise mental health awareness and destigmatize discussions surrounding self-harm and suicide within our communities.

In the subsequent chapters, we will further explore strategies for crisis intervention, risk assessment, and suicide prevention, emphasising the importance of collaborative efforts in promoting mental well-being.

Seeking Help for Individuals Struggling with Self-Harm or Suicidal Thoughts

Recognising the signs of self-harm or suicidal ideation is the first step towards seeking appropriate help and support for individuals in distress. Knowing when and how to intervene effectively can make a significant difference in promoting mental health and preventing crises.

When to Seek Help:

Immediate Danger: If an individual expresses immediate plans or intent to harm themselves or others, seek emergency assistance without delay. Call emergency services (911 or equivalent) or accompany them to the nearest hospital emergency department.

Visible Signs of Self-Harm: If you notice physical signs of self-harm (e.g., cuts, bruises, burns) or suspect that an individual is engaging in self-harm behaviours, encourage them to seek professional help.

Verbal Expressions of Distress: Pay attention to verbal cues indicating thoughts of suicide or hopelessness. Take statements about self-harm seriously and initiate supportive conversations.

Behavioural Changes: Significant changes in behaviour, mood, or social interactions may signal underlying emotional distress requiring intervention.

How to Seek Help:

Encourage Open Communication:

Approach the individual with empathy and compassion.

Express concern and willingness to listen without judgment.

Create a safe and supportive environment for open dialogue.

Connect with Mental Health Professionals:

Encourage the individual to schedule an appointment with a licensed therapist, counsellor, or psychiatrist specialising in mental health and suicide prevention.

Assist in researching local mental health resources and crisis intervention services.

Utilize Crisis Hotlines:

Provide access to crisis hotlines and suicide prevention helplines for immediate support and guidance.

Offer to make the call together or assist in finding online chat services for confidential communication.

Seek Community Support:

Encourage involvement in peer support groups, community organisations, or religious/spiritual communities offering mental health resources and support networks.

Develop a Safety Plan:

Collaborate with mental health professionals to develop a personalised safety plan addressing triggers, coping strategies, and emergency contacts.

Ensure access to crisis intervention resources and emergency services.

Remove Access to Means:

Minimise access to lethal means of self-harm, such as medications, sharp objects, or firearms, to reduce immediate risk.

Provide Ongoing Support:

Offer ongoing emotional support and follow-up care to reinforce recovery and resilience.

Encourage engagement in therapeutic interventions and adherence to treatment plans.

When to Involve Emergency Services:

If an individual is actively harming themselves or expressing imminent plans for suicide.

If the individual is unable to ensure their safety or requires immediate medical attention.

Remember:

Take all signs of distress seriously and prioritise safety above all else.

Foster open communication and empower individuals to seek help without shame or stigma.

Collaborate with mental health professionals, crisis intervention teams, and support networks to provide comprehensive care and promote recovery.

By taking proactive steps to seek help and support for individuals struggling with self-harm or suicidal thoughts, we can play a critical role in saving lives and promoting mental well-being within our communities.

In the subsequent chapters, we will continue to explore strategies for crisis intervention, suicide prevention, and building resilience among individuals at risk.

5. Impact of Suicide on Loved Ones: Exploring the Unique Challenges of Bereavement

The aftermath of a suicide death is profoundly devastating and can have lasting emotional, psychological, and social repercussions on surviving loved ones. Exploring the unique challenges of bereavement after suicide is essential for understanding grief reactions and facilitating healing within affected communities.

Understanding the Impact:

Shock and Disbelief:

Survivors often experience initial shock and disbelief upon learning about the suicide death of a loved one. The sudden and unexpected nature of suicide can make acceptance and understanding difficult.

Intense Emotional Responses:

Bereaved individuals may experience a range of intense emotions, including profound sadness, anger, guilt, shame, and profound loss. The complex emotions associated with suicide bereavement can be overwhelming and persistent.

Stigma and Shame:

Suicide remains highly stigmatised in many societies, leading to feelings of shame, isolation, and social judgment for surviving family members and friends.

Unanswered Questions and Guilt:

Survivors often grapple with unanswered questions about why the suicide occurred and whether they could have done more to prevent it. Feelings of guilt and self-blame are common and can complicate the grieving process.

Complicated Grief Reactions:

Suicide bereavement is associated with higher rates of complicated grief reactions, including prolonged mourning, intrusive thoughts, and difficulty finding closure.

Unique Challenges of Suicide Bereavement:

Social Isolation:

Survivors may face social withdrawal and isolation due to stigma surrounding suicide, leading to strained relationships and reduced social support.

Ambiguous Loss:

Suicide often leaves survivors with feelings of unresolved grief and ambiguous loss, as they grapple with the absence of closure and understanding.

Coping with Trauma:

Witnessing or discovering the aftermath of a suicide can be traumatic for survivors, exacerbating feelings of distress and emotional upheaval.

Impact on Children and Family Dynamics:

Children and family members may struggle to process the loss of a loved one to suicide, leading to disruptions in family dynamics and challenges in parenting.

Facilitating Healing and Support:

Open Dialogue and Supportive Communities:

Encourage open dialogue about suicide bereavement to reduce stigma and foster supportive communities for survivors.

Facilitate peer support groups, therapy sessions, and community initiatives to provide validation and connection for grieving individuals.

Professional Counselling and Therapy:

Provide access to specialised grief counselling and therapy for survivors of suicide, addressing complex emotions and facilitating coping strategies.

Educational Initiatives:

Promote education and awareness about suicide bereavement within schools, workplaces, and community settings to reduce stigma and enhance empathy.

Resilience and Coping Strategies:

Empower survivors with resilience-building strategies and self-care practices to navigate the challenges of suicide bereavement and promote emotional healing.

By exploring the unique challenges of suicide bereavement and fostering supportive interventions, we can promote understanding, reduce stigma, and facilitate healing within communities impacted by suicide loss.

In the subsequent chapters, we will look deeper into strategies for coping with suicide bereavement, fostering resilience, and promoting post intervention initiatives to support survivors on their journey toward healing.

Coping with the Emotional Aftermath and Social Stigma

The emotional aftermath of suicide loss is uniquely challenging, often compounded by societal stigma and misconceptions surrounding mental health and suicide. Coping with grief and navigating social dynamics requires resilience, support, and compassionate understanding.

Understanding the Emotional Aftermath:

1. **Intense Grief and Loss:**

Survivors of suicide loss experience profound grief and loss, characterised by waves of intense sadness, despair, and emotional upheaval.

Coping with the sudden and unexpected nature of suicide can complicate mourning and extend the grieving process.

2. **Guilt and Self-Blame:**

Survivors often grapple with feelings of guilt, self-blame, and unanswered questions about the circumstances leading to the suicide. They may question their ability to recognise warning signs or prevent the tragedy.

3. **Anger and Resentment:**

Feelings of anger and resentment towards the deceased, mental health professionals, or societal institutions may arise as survivors navigate complex emotions.

4. **Trauma and Intrusive Thoughts:**

Witnessing or discovering the aftermath of a suicide can be traumatic, leading to intrusive thoughts, nightmares, and heightened anxiety.

Coping Strategies for Emotional Healing:

1. **Seeking Professional Support:**

Engage in grief counselling, therapy, or support groups specifically tailored for suicide bereavement. Professional guidance can provide validation, coping strategies, and emotional processing.

2. **Expressive Outlets:**

Explore creative outlets such as writing, art, or music to express emotions and navigate the complexities of grief.

3. **Mindfulness and Self-Care:**

Practice mindfulness meditation, yoga, or relaxation techniques to manage stress and promote emotional well-being.

Prioritise self-care activities that nurture physical, emotional, and spiritual health.

4. **Connecting with Support Networks:**

Lean on trusted friends, family members, or peer support groups who can offer empathy, companionship, and understanding.

Participate in community events or initiatives that promote mental health awareness and suicide prevention.

Navigating Social Stigma:

1. **Addressing Misconceptions:**

Challenge societal misconceptions about suicide and mental health by engaging in open dialogue and sharing personal experiences.

Educate others about the complexities of suicide bereavement and the importance of empathy and support.

2. **Creating Safe Spaces:**

Advocate for stigma-free environments within workplaces, schools, and communities to promote inclusivity and reduce shame associated with suicide loss.

3. **Setting Boundaries:**

Establish boundaries with individuals who perpetuate stigma or insensitivity towards suicide bereavement.

Surround yourself with supportive individuals who prioritise understanding and empathy.

4. **Redefining Narratives:**

Encourage storytelling and narrative-sharing to redefine societal narratives around suicide loss and honour the memories of loved ones.

Embracing Resilience and Healing:

1. **Honouring Memories:**

Create meaningful rituals, memorials, or tribute projects to celebrate the life and legacy of the deceased.

Participate in suicide prevention efforts or advocacy initiatives as a way to channel grief into positive action.

2. **Embracing Growth and Transformation:**

Embrace personal growth and transformation through self-reflection, self-compassion, and embracing new perspectives on life.

Recognise the strength and resilience inherent in the journey of suicide bereavement.

By actively coping with the emotional aftermath of suicide and challenging social stigma, survivors can cultivate resilience, foster healing, and contribute to meaningful change within their communities.

In the subsequent chapters, we will continue to explore practical coping strategies, resilience-building techniques, and advocacy initiatives to support individuals navigating the complexities of suicide bereavement.

Supporting Family and Friends Affected by Suicide Loss

Suicide loss profoundly impacts the lives of family members and friends, creating unique challenges and emotional upheaval. Providing compassionate support and fostering resilience within affected communities is essential for healing and navigating the complexities of grief.

Understanding the Impact on Family and Friends:

1. **Profound Grief and Loss:**

Family members and friends experience profound grief and loss following a suicide death, characterised by intense emotions, disbelief, and emotional turmoil.

The sudden and unexpected nature of suicide can complicate mourning and extend the grieving process.

2. **Complex Emotions:**

Survivors grapple with a range of complex emotions, including sadness, anger, guilt, shame, and profound emptiness.

Feelings of confusion and disbelief may arise as loved ones struggle to comprehend the reasons behind the suicide.

3. **Stigma and Social Isolation:**

Survivors often face societal stigma and misconceptions surrounding suicide, leading to feelings of shame, isolation, and judgment.

Social withdrawal and strained relationships may result from the challenges of navigating grief in the aftermath of suicide.

Practical Strategies for Providing Support:

1.   **Offering Compassionate Presence:**

Be present and available to listen without judgment or expectation. Allow survivors to express their emotions and share their experiences openly.

2.   **Validating Feelings and Experiences:**

Validate the range of emotions experienced by survivors, acknowledging the complexity of grief and loss following suicide.

Avoid minimising or dismissing feelings of guilt, anger, or confusion.

3.   **Encouraging Open Communication:**

Foster open dialogue about suicide loss within families and friend circles, emphasising empathy, understanding, and mutual support.

Facilitate honest conversations about coping strategies, emotional processing, and self-care.

4.   **Connecting with Resources:**

Provide information about grief counselling, support groups, and community resources specialising in suicide bereavement.

Assist in researching local mental health services and crisis intervention helplines.

5.   **Creating Rituals and Memorials:**

Encourage survivors to create meaningful rituals, memorials, or tribute projects honouring the memory of the deceased.

Participate in commemorative events or suicide prevention initiatives as a way to channel grief into positive action.

Navigating Challenges and Building Resilience:

1. **Understanding Individual Needs:**

Recognise that grief reactions vary among individuals and families. Respect individual coping styles and timelines for healing.

2. **Promoting Self-Care and Well-Being:**

Emphasise the importance of self-care practices, including mindfulness, exercise, and relaxation techniques, to promote emotional well-being.

Encourage healthy coping strategies and adaptive responses to grief-related challenges.

3. **Advocating for Change:**

Engage in advocacy efforts to challenge stigma, raise awareness about suicide prevention, and promote access to mental health resources within communities.

Embracing Collective Healing and Resilience:

1. **Building Support Networks:**

Facilitate connections with other suicide loss survivors and peer support groups to foster solidarity and mutual understanding.

Encourage shared experiences and collaborative efforts towards healing and resilience.

2. **Honouring Memories and Legacies:**

Create opportunities to honour the memories and legacies of the deceased through storytelling, creative expression, and acts of remembrance.

Embrace resilience as a collective journey of healing and transformation within affected families and communities.

By providing compassionate support, fostering open communication, and advocating for systemic change, we can empower family members and friends affected by suicide loss to navigate grief and build resilience on their healing journeys.

In the subsequent chapters, we will continue to explore practical strategies, therapeutic interventions, and community initiatives aimed at supporting individuals and communities impacted by suicide bereavement.

6. Coping Strategies for Self-Harm and Emotional Distress: Alternative Mechanisms

Navigating emotional distress and managing urges to self-harm require proactive coping strategies and healthy alternatives. Exploring alternative coping mechanisms empowers individuals to address underlying emotions and develop resilience in times of distress.

Understanding the Cycle of Self-Harm:

1. **Triggers and Emotional Responses:**

Self-harm often serves as a maladaptive coping mechanism in response to overwhelming emotions, stress, or trauma.

Identifying triggers and emotional cues that precede self-harm behaviours is crucial for developing effective coping strategies.

2. **Emotional Regulation and Coping Styles:**

Individuals may engage in self-harm to regulate intense emotions, numb emotional pain, or seek temporary relief from distressing thoughts.

Alternative Coping Mechanisms:

1. **Mindfulness and Relaxation Techniques:**

Practice mindfulness meditation, deep breathing exercises, or progressive muscle relaxation to manage stress and promote emotional regulation.

Explore yoga, tai chi, or guided imagery to cultivate a sense of calmness and inner peace.

2. **Creative Outlets:**

Engage in creative activities such as drawing, painting, writing, or playing musical instruments as a means of self-expression and emotional release.

Use art therapy techniques to externalise emotions and process underlying feelings in a safe and constructive manner.

3. **Physical Activities:**

Channel emotional energy into physical activities such as jogging, dancing, or practicing martial arts to release tension and boost endorphins.

Incorporate regular exercise routines into daily life to promote overall well-being and stress reduction.

4. **Social Connection and Support:**

Reach out to trusted friends, family members, or support networks for companionship, empathy, and understanding during times of distress.

Participate in group activities, volunteer work, or community initiatives to foster social connections and combat feelings of isolation.

5. **Cognitive-Behavioural Techniques:**

Implement cognitive-behavioural strategies, such as cognitive restructuring and thought challenging, to modify negative thought patterns and enhance self-awareness.

Practice self-compassion and self-validation to counteract feelings of guilt or self-blame associated with self-harm urges.

6. **Distraction and Grounding Techniques:**

Employ distraction techniques, such as engaging in hobbies, solving puzzles, or watching movies, to divert attention away from self-harm urges.

Use grounding exercises, such as sensory awareness or mindfulness of the present moment, to stay anchored and centred during distressing episodes.

Building Resilience and Long-Term Recovery:

1. **Self-Care Practices:**

Prioritise self-care activities, including adequate sleep, nutrition, and hydration, to support overall physical and emotional well-being.

Establish healthy routines and self-care rituals to promote stability and resilience in daily life.

2. **Professional Support and Therapy:**

Seek professional help from mental health professionals specialising in dialectical behaviour therapy (DBT), cognitive-behavioural therapy (CBT), or trauma-focused interventions.

Collaborate with therapists to develop personalised coping strategies and crisis management plans tailored to individual needs.

3. **Progressive Goals and Self-Empowerment:**

Set achievable goals and milestones to celebrate progress and foster a sense of accomplishment.

Cultivate self-empowerment through positive affirmations, self-reflection, and active participation in recovery-oriented activities.

By exploring alternative coping mechanisms, individuals can replace self-harm behaviours with adaptive strategies that promote emotional regulation, self-expression, and long-term recovery. It's essential to prioritise self-awareness, self-care, and proactive intervention in managing emotional distress effectively.

In the subsequent chapters, we will continue to explore evidence-based approaches, therapeutic interventions, and self-help techniques aimed at fostering resilience and promoting healthy coping strategies for individuals struggling with self-harm urges.

Developing Healthy Coping Skills and Emotional Regulation Techniques

Effective emotional regulation and healthy coping skills are essential for navigating life's challenges and managing stress without resorting to harmful behaviours like self-harm. Building a toolbox of adaptive strategies empowers individuals to cope with distressing emotions and promote overall well-being.

Understanding Emotional Regulation:

1. **Awareness of Emotional Triggers:**

Recognise personal triggers that evoke strong emotional responses, such as stress, anxiety, trauma reminders, or interpersonal conflicts.

Develop self-awareness of emotional states and associated physiological reactions (e.g., increased heart rate, muscle tension).

2. **Coping Strategies for Emotional Regulation:**

Implement adaptive coping strategies to modulate emotional responses and promote self-regulation in challenging situations.

Cultivate mindfulness and emotional awareness to observe, acknowledge, and respond to emotions without judgment.

Healthy Coping Skills:

1. **Mindfulness and Meditation:**

Practice mindfulness meditation to cultivate present-moment awareness and detach from distressing thoughts and emotions.

Engage in mindful activities such as mindful eating, walking, or body scanning to enhance emotional regulation.

2. **Stress Management Techniques:**

Learn stress reduction techniques, including deep breathing exercises, progressive muscle relaxation, or guided imagery, to alleviate tension and promote relaxation.

Incorporate regular physical exercise, such as yoga, jogging, or dancing, to release endorphins and reduce stress levels.

3. **Effective Communication:**

Develop assertive communication skills to express emotions, set boundaries, and address interpersonal conflicts constructively.

Seek support from trusted individuals and communicate openly about emotional struggles and coping needs.

4. **Problem-Solving and Resilience-Building:**

Enhance problem-solving skills by breaking down challenges into manageable steps and identifying practical solutions.

Foster resilience through adaptive coping strategies, positive reframing, and focusing on strengths and personal growth.

5. **Creative Expression and Self-Discovery:**

Explore creative outlets such as art therapy, journaling, music, or poetry to express emotions and promote self-discovery.

Use creative activities as a means of processing emotions, reducing anxiety, and fostering emotional resilience.

Developing Effective Coping Strategies:

1. **Identifying Personal Coping Preferences:**

Explore a range of coping techniques to identify preferred strategies that resonate with individual needs and preferences.

Experiment with different techniques and adapt them to specific situations and emotional states.

2. **Building Adaptive Coping Skills:**

Engage in proactive coping behaviours that promote emotional regulation and reduce reliance on maladaptive coping mechanisms (e.g., self-harm, substance use).

Foster self-compassion and self-acceptance while developing new coping skills and adapting to setbacks.

3. **Seeking Professional Guidance:**

Consult mental health professionals, counsellors, or therapists for personalised guidance and support in developing healthy coping skills.

Participate in therapy modalities such as cognitive-behavioural therapy (CBT), dialectical behaviour therapy (DBT), or acceptance and commitment therapy (ACT) to enhance emotional regulation.

Integrating Coping Skills into Daily Life:

1. **Consistent Practice and Routine:**

Incorporate coping skills into daily routines to reinforce positive habits and promote emotional resilience over time.

Set reminders or schedule designated times for practicing coping techniques to prioritise self-care and emotional well-being.

2. **Adapting to Changing Needs:**

Remain flexible and adaptive in refining coping strategies based on evolving emotional needs and life circumstances.

Recognise the importance of ongoing self-care and proactive coping to maintain emotional balance and prevent relapse.

By developing healthy coping skills and mastering emotional regulation techniques, individuals can cultivate resilience, manage stress effectively, and navigate emotional challenges with greater confidence and self-awareness.

In the subsequent chapters, we will continue to explore practical strategies, therapeutic interventions, and resilience-building techniques aimed at promoting emotional well-being and supporting individuals on their journey towards recovery.

The Role of Therapy and Professional Support in Recovery from Self-Harm

Therapy and professional support play a pivotal role in the recovery journey for individuals struggling with self-harm behaviours. Accessing specialised interventions and therapeutic modalities empowers individuals to address underlying issues, develop healthy coping strategies, and foster long-term recovery.

Understanding the Impact of Self-Harm:

1. **Complex Underlying Factors:**

Self-harm often stems from complex psychological, emotional, and interpersonal factors, including trauma, stress, low self-esteem, and difficulty managing emotions.

Individuals may use self-harm as a maladaptive coping mechanism to regulate emotions, numb emotional pain, or communicate distress.

2. **Cycle of Self-Harm and Emotional Distress:**

Engaging in self-harm can perpetuate a cycle of shame, guilt, and emotional distress, reinforcing the need for specialised intervention and support.

The Role of Therapy in Recovery:

1. **Behavioural Therapies:**

Cognitive-Behavioural Therapy (CBT): CBT focuses on identifying and challenging negative thought patterns and behaviours associated with self-harm. It helps individuals develop adaptive coping skills and alternative strategies to manage distress.

Dialectical Behaviour Therapy (DBT): DBT integrates mindfulness, emotion regulation, distress tolerance, and interpersonal skills training to address self-harm behaviours. It emphasises validation, acceptance, and building a life worth living.

2. Trauma-Informed Approaches:

Trauma-Focused Therapy: For individuals with a history of trauma, trauma-focused therapy helps process traumatic experiences, reduce triggers, and develop effective coping mechanisms.

Eye Movement Desensitization and Reprocessing (EMDR): EMDR targets distressing memories and associated beliefs to promote emotional healing and adaptive resolution of trauma.

3. Interpersonal Therapy:

Interpersonal therapy focuses on improving interpersonal relationships, communication skills, and conflict resolution to address underlying emotional triggers for self-harm.

4. Family Therapy and Support:

Family therapy involves family members in the recovery process, fostering understanding, communication, and support within the family system.

Collaborative approaches help address family dynamics, enhance coping strategies, and promote shared responsibility in supporting recovery.

Professional Support in Recovery:

1. **Comprehensive Assessment and Treatment Planning:**

Mental health professionals conduct comprehensive assessments to understand individual needs, risk factors, and treatment goals.

Treatment plans are tailored to address underlying issues, prioritise safety, and promote holistic recovery.

2. **Skill-Building and Coping Strategies:**

Therapists teach coping skills, emotion regulation techniques, and stress management strategies to empower individuals in managing emotional distress and reducing self-harm urges.

Skills training promotes adaptive responses to triggers and enhances resilience in challenging situations.

3. **Addressing Underlying Issues:**

Therapy sessions explore underlying issues contributing to self-harm behaviours, including trauma, depression, anxiety, or interpersonal difficulties.

Therapists provide validation, empathy, and non-judgmental support to facilitate emotional processing and healing.

Long-Term Recovery and Relapse Prevention:

1. **Continuity of Care and Follow-Up:**

Ongoing therapy and follow-up appointments ensure continuity of care, monitor progress, and address emerging challenges in recovery.

Therapists collaborate with individuals to develop relapse prevention plans and adaptive coping strategies for sustaining recovery.

2. **Integration of Self-Care Practices:**

Therapists emphasise self-care practices, healthy lifestyle habits, and community support networks to promote sustained well-being and prevent relapse.

Peer support groups and community resources complement professional therapy by fostering connection, understanding, and mutual support.

Empowering Recovery and Personal Growth:

1. **Self-Exploration and Personal Development:**

Therapy encourages self-exploration, self-awareness, and personal growth by fostering insights, resilience, and adaptive coping skills.

Individuals develop a sense of agency, autonomy, and empowerment in navigating recovery and building a meaningful life beyond self-harm.

2. **Reducing Stigma and Promoting Awareness:**

Therapy challenges stigma surrounding mental health and self-harm, promoting empathy, understanding, and destigmatisation within communities.

Increased awareness and advocacy efforts contribute to systemic changes that prioritise mental health support and suicide prevention.

By recognising the integral role of therapy and professional support in recovery from self-harm, individuals can access specialized interventions, develop effective coping strategies, and embark on a journey towards healing, resilience, and personal transformation.

In the subsequent chapters, we will continue to explore recovery-oriented approaches, therapeutic modalities, and community initiatives aimed at promoting mental well-being and supporting individuals in overcoming self-harm behaviours.

7. Supporting Those Affected by Suicide: Providing Practical Guidance for Caregivers and Support Networks

Supporting individuals affected by suicide requires compassion, empathy, and practical strategies to navigate grief, trauma, and emotional distress. Caregivers and support networks play a crucial role in fostering healing and resilience within affected communities.

Understanding the Impact of Suicide:

1. **Complex Grief Reactions:**

Survivors of suicide loss experience a range of complex grief reactions, including shock, disbelief, intense sadness, anger, guilt, and emotional turmoil.

Recognise the unique challenges of suicide bereavement, such as stigma, social isolation, and unresolved questions surrounding the suicide.

2. **Trauma and Emotional Distress:**

Suicide can be traumatic for surviving family members and friends, leading to heightened emotional distress, intrusive thoughts, and challenges in coping with loss.

Providing Practical Guidance for Caregivers and Support Networks:

1. **Establishing Open Communication:**

Encourage open dialogue and communication within support networks, allowing individuals to express emotions, share experiences, and seek guidance without judgment.

Foster a safe and supportive environment that promotes empathy, understanding, and mutual support.

2. **Offering Emotional Support:**

Provide compassionate and non-judgmental emotional support to individuals affected by suicide, acknowledging their pain and validating their experiences.

Listen actively, show empathy, and offer reassurance while respecting individual coping styles and emotional needs.

3. **Educating on Grief and Coping Strategies:**

Educate caregivers and support networks about the complexities of grief after suicide loss, emphasising the importance of self-care, resilience-building, and adaptive coping strategies.

Share information about common grief reactions, triggers, and healthy ways to navigate emotional distress.

4. **Practical Assistance and Resource Navigation:**

Assist caregivers in navigating practical challenges associated with suicide bereavement, such as funeral arrangements, legal matters, and accessing mental health resources.

Provide information about grief counselling, support groups, crisis helplines, and community services available for individuals affected by suicide.

5. **Promoting Self-Care and Well-Being:**

Encourage caregivers and support networks to prioritise self-care practices, including adequate rest, nutrition, exercise, and stress management.

Emphasise the importance of seeking professional help or therapy if needed to process grief and cope with emotional challenges.

Addressing Stigma and Building Resilience:

1. **Challenging Stigma and Misconceptions:**

Advocate for destigmatisation of suicide and mental health within communities, promoting empathy, understanding, and supportive attitudes towards survivors.

Educate others about suicide prevention, risk factors, and the impact of stigma on individuals affected by suicide loss.

2. **Building Resilient Communities:**

Foster community-based initiatives, support groups, and peer networks to promote solidarity, resilience, and mutual support among individuals affected by suicide.

Collaborate with local organisations, schools, and healthcare providers to enhance suicide prevention efforts and promote mental health awareness.

Encouraging Healing and Meaning-Making:

1. **Honouring Memories and Legacies:**

Facilitate meaningful rituals, memorials, or commemorative events to honour the lives and legacies of those lost to suicide.

Encourage storytelling, creative expression, and acts of remembrance to promote healing and meaning-making within affected communities.

2. **Facilitating Recovery-Oriented Approaches:**

Support individuals in their journey towards recovery by fostering hope, resilience, and adaptive coping skills.

Promote recovery-oriented approaches that prioritise empowerment, self-determination, and personal growth after suicide loss.

By providing practical guidance, emotional support, and advocacy efforts, caregivers and support networks can play a vital role in promoting healing, resilience, and community solidarity among individuals affected by suicide.

In the subsequent chapters, we will continue to explore practical strategies, community interventions, and advocacy initiatives aimed at supporting individuals and communities impacted by suicide loss.

How to Offer Empathetic and Non-Judgmental Support to Individuals Affected by Suicide

Providing empathetic and non-judgmental support is essential in assisting individuals affected by suicide to navigate grief, trauma, and emotional distress. Building genuine connections and fostering understanding can promote healing and resilience within affected communities.

Principles of Empathetic Support:

1. **Active Listening:**

Practice active listening by giving your full attention to the individual, maintaining eye contact, and showing genuine interest in their experiences.

Validate emotions and reflect back what you hear to demonstrate understanding and empathy.

2. **Cultivating Empathy:**

Put yourself in the individual's shoes, acknowledging their pain, struggles, and unique grief journey.

Show empathy through compassionate responses, gestures of kindness, and non-verbal cues that convey understanding and care.

Key Strategies for Non-Judgmental Support:

1. **Avoiding Assumptions and Preconceptions:**

Approach conversations with an open mind and refrain from making assumptions about the individual's feelings, behaviours, or experiences.

Suspend judgment and focus on listening without imposing personal beliefs or values.

2. **Respecting Individual Coping Styles:**

Recognise that individuals may cope with grief and trauma in different ways. Respect their coping strategies and emotional responses without criticism or interference.

Offer support tailored to their needs and preferences, honouring their autonomy and personal agency.

Practical Tips for Offering Support:

1. **Create Safe and Supportive Spaces:**

Foster environments where individuals feel safe, accepted, and free to express themselves without fear of judgment or stigma.

Respect confidentiality and privacy while maintaining boundaries and ethical considerations.

2. **Validate Feelings and Experiences:**

Validate the individual's emotions, experiences, and reactions without minimising or dismissing their pain.

Use validating statements such as "I hear you," "It's okay to feel this way," or "You are not alone."

3. **Ask Open-Ended Questions:**

Encourage open dialogue and exploration of feelings by asking open-ended questions that invite reflection and deeper sharing.

Avoid probing or intrusive questions and allow the individual to share at their own pace.

4. **Express Empathy Through Words and Actions:**

Offer verbal expressions of empathy, such as "I'm here for you," "I care about you," or "You matter."

Show empathy through supportive actions, such as offering practical assistance, running errands, or providing companionship.

Building Trust and Connection:

1. **Demonstrate Consistency and Reliability:**

Build trust over time by demonstrating consistency, reliability, and follow-through in your support efforts.

Honour commitments and be present during challenging moments without judgment or withdrawal.

2. **Respecting Boundaries and Self-Determination:**

Respect the individual's boundaries, autonomy, and right to make decisions about their own healing journey.

Offer support as a facilitator of empowerment and self-determination, respecting their choices and preferences.

Promoting Healing and Resilience:

1. **Encouraging Help-Seeking Behaviours:**

Normalise help-seeking behaviours and encourage individuals to access professional support, counselling, or therapy as needed.

Provide information about mental health resources, crisis helplines, and support groups available for individuals affected by suicide.

2. **Advocating for Awareness and destigmatisation:**

Advocate for awareness and destigmatisation of suicide and mental health within communities, promoting empathy, understanding, and supportive attitudes.

Challenge societal misconceptions and contribute to creating inclusive, compassionate environments for those affected by suicide.

By offering empathetic and non-judgmental support, individuals can foster healing, promote resilience, and empower individuals affected by suicide to navigate their grief journey with dignity, compassion, and hope.

In the subsequent chapters, we will continue to explore practical strategies, communication techniques, and community initiatives aimed at supporting individuals and communities impacted by suicide.

8. Navigating Grief and Healing: Understanding the Stages of Grief and the Grieving Process after Suicide Loss

Grief following a suicide loss is a complex and deeply personal experience, characterised by intense emotions, cognitive struggles, and existential questions. Understanding the stages of grief and the dynamics of the grieving process can empower individuals to navigate their healing journey with compassion and resilience.

Understanding the Stages of Grief:

Grief is not a linear process but rather a series of emotional and psychological stages that individuals may cycle through non-sequentially. The stages of grief commonly associated with loss, including suicide loss, include:

1. **Shock and Denial:**

Initially, individuals may experience shock and disbelief, struggling to comprehend the reality of the loss.

Denial serves as a protective mechanism, allowing individuals to process overwhelming emotions gradually.

2. **Anger and Guilt:**

As reality sets in, survivors may experience intense anger directed towards the deceased, oneself, or others perceived to be involved.

Feelings of guilt and self-blame are common, as individuals grapple with unanswered questions and perceived shortcomings.

3. **Bargaining and Searching for Meaning:**

Grieving individuals may engage in bargaining, attempting to negotiate with a higher power or make sense of the loss through spiritual or existential inquiries.

The search for meaning involves seeking understanding, purpose, or significance in the midst of profound loss.

4. **Depression and Emotional Withdrawal:**

Deep sadness, despair, and emotional withdrawal may characterize this stage, as individuals confront the full weight of their loss.

Symptoms of depression, such as feelings of emptiness, lethargy, and social withdrawal, may intensify during this phase.

5. **Acceptance and Integration:**

Over time, individuals gradually come to accept the reality of the loss and integrate it into their sense of self and life narrative.

Acceptance does not signify the absence of grief but rather a transformative process of adaptation and emotional reconciliation.

The Dynamics of Grieving Process after Suicide Loss:

1. **Complex Grief Reactions:**

Suicide loss can trigger complex grief reactions, including trauma, survivor guilt, and existential crises.

Individuals may struggle with intrusive thoughts, survivor's guilt, and existential questions surrounding the reasons behind the suicide.

2. **Social and Cultural Influences:**

Grieving processes are influenced by social norms, cultural beliefs, and familial dynamics that shape the expression and management of grief.

Stigma and societal misconceptions surrounding suicide may complicate the grieving process and impact social support networks.

Practical Strategies for Navigating Grief and Healing:

1. **Seeking Professional Support:**

Access grief counselling, therapy, or support groups specialising in suicide bereavement to process emotions, address trauma and develop coping strategies.

Engage in trauma-informed therapies, such as EMDR or narrative therapy, to navigate complex grief reactions and promote emotional healing.

2. **Embracing Self-Care and Compassion:**

Prioritise self-care practices, including rest, nutrition, exercise, and mindfulness, to support emotional well-being during grief.

Practice self-compassion and self-kindness, acknowledging the challenges of grief and allowing oneself space for healing.

3. **Fostering Supportive Connections:**

Lean on supportive relationships, family members, friends, or peer support groups to share experiences, receive validation, and foster mutual understanding.

Engage in rituals, commemorative activities, or creative expressions to honour the memory of the deceased and promote healing.

4. **Exploring Meaning-Making and Legacy:**

Explore existential questions and engage in meaning-making activities to derive purpose and significance from the loss.

Reflect on the legacy of the deceased and ways to honour their memory through advocacy, storytelling, or community initiatives.

Promoting Resilience and Growth:

1. **Embracing Adaptive Coping Strategies:**

Develop adaptive coping strategies, such as mindfulness, cognitive reframing, and expressive arts, to manage grief-related distress and foster resilience.

Set realistic goals and milestones to celebrate progress and promote a sense of agency in the healing journey.

2. **Advocating for Mental Health Awareness:**

Advocate for mental health awareness, suicide prevention initiatives, and destigmatisation efforts within communities to promote empathy, understanding, and support.

Participate in advocacy projects or community outreach activities to raise awareness about suicide bereavement and promote healing-centred approaches.

By understanding the stages of grief and the dynamics of the grieving process after suicide loss, individuals can navigate their healing journey with compassion, resilience, and a sense of purpose. Each person's grief experience is unique, and embracing supportive resources and meaningful connections can facilitate emotional healing and promote growth in the aftermath of loss.

In the subsequent chapters, we will continue to explore practical strategies, therapeutic interventions, and community initiatives aimed at supporting individuals and communities impacted by suicide loss.

Finding Meaning and Support in the Journey of Healing

Navigating the journey of healing after experiencing suicide loss involves seeking meaning, fostering resilience, and accessing supportive resources to promote emotional well-being and personal growth. Finding purpose and support within the healing process can empower individuals to honour their grief, cultivate resilience, and embrace life with renewed meaning.

Exploring Meaning-Making:

1. **Seeking Understanding and Acceptance:**

Engage in introspection and self-reflection to explore existential questions and find personal meaning in the aftermath of suicide loss.

Embrace acceptance of the loss while acknowledging the profound impact it has had on personal identity and life narratives.

2. **Connecting with Shared Experiences:**

Seek solace and validation through connecting with others who have experienced similar losses, fostering empathy, understanding, and mutual support.

Participate in peer support groups, online forums, or community initiatives that promote solidarity and shared healing experiences.

Fostering Resilience and Growth:

1. **Cultivating Adaptive Coping Strategies:**

Develop adaptive coping strategies, such as mindfulness, meditation, creative expression, and physical activity, to manage grief-related distress and promote resilience.

Embrace self-care practices that prioritise emotional well-being, nurture self-compassion, and foster a sense of agency in the healing journey.

2. Embracing Personal Growth and Transformation:

Embrace opportunities for personal growth and transformation by channelling grief into meaningful pursuits, creative endeavours, or advocacy initiatives.

Set intentions for growth, self-discovery, and purposeful living that honour the memory of the deceased and promote healing-centred approaches.

Accessing Supportive Resources:

1. Professional Counselling and Therapy:

Seek specialised grief counselling, therapy, or support from mental health professionals trained in trauma-informed approaches and suicide bereavement.

Engage in therapies, such as narrative therapy, EMDR, or group counselling, to process emotions, address trauma, and navigate complex grief reactions.

2. Community and Peer Support Networks:

Leverage community resources, peer support networks, and local organisations specializing in suicide bereavement to access compassionate support and practical guidance.

Participate in commemorative events, memorial services, or awareness campaigns that promote healing and destigmatisation within communities.

Honouring the Memory and Legacy:

1. **Creating Meaningful Rituals and Commemorative Activities:**

Design rituals, ceremonies, or commemorative activities that honour the memory and legacy of the deceased, fostering connections and promoting healing.

Engage in storytelling, creative expressions, or acts of remembrance that celebrate the life and impact of the loved one lost to suicide.

2. **Advocacy and Community Engagement:**

Advocate for mental health awareness, suicide prevention initiatives, and destigmatisation efforts within communities to promote empathy, understanding, and support.

Engage in advocacy projects, volunteer opportunities, or grassroots campaigns that contribute to systemic changes and promote healing-centred approaches.

Embracing Hope and Renewed Purpose:

1. **Cultivating Hope and Resilience:**

Embrace hope as a guiding force in the healing journey, recognising the potential for growth, resilience, and renewed purpose after experiencing suicide loss.

Foster a sense of resilience by embracing adaptive strategies, nurturing supportive relationships, and actively participating in healing-centred activities.

2. **Continuing the Journey of Healing:**

Embrace the journey of healing as an ongoing process of self-discovery, growth, and integration of loss into personal narratives.

Celebrate milestones, acknowledge progress, and honour the resilience demonstrated throughout the healing journey.

By finding meaning, fostering resilience, and accessing supportive resources within the journey of healing, individuals can navigate the complexities of grief after suicide loss with compassion, purpose, and hope. Each person's healing journey is unique, and embracing supportive connections and meaningful experiences can promote emotional well-being and facilitate transformative growth.

In the subsequent chapters, we will continue to explore practical strategies, therapeutic interventions, and community initiatives aimed at supporting individuals and communities impacted by suicide loss.

Accessing Grief Support Services and Resources in Ireland and the UK

Navigating grief after experiencing suicide loss can be a challenging and complex journey. Accessing specialised grief support services and resources tailored to the needs of individuals and families affected by suicide can facilitate healing, promote resilience, and foster meaningful connections within the community.

Grief Support Services in Ireland:

1. **Pieta House:**

    Pieta House is a leading organisation in Ireland dedicated to providing free therapy and support to individuals experiencing suicidal ideation, self-harm, and those bereaved by suicide.

    Services offered include one-to-one counselling, family support sessions, bereavement support groups, and crisis intervention.

2. **Samaritans Ireland:**

    Samaritans Ireland offers confidential emotional support to individuals in distress, including those affected by suicide loss.

    The helpline (116 123) operates 24/7, providing a listening ear, emotional support, and crisis intervention for individuals experiencing grief or emotional distress.

3. **Aware:**

    Aware is a mental health organisation in Ireland that provides support and information for individuals affected by depression, anxiety, and related mood disorders.

Aware offers support groups, online resources, and educational programs that may be beneficial for individuals navigating grief after suicide loss.

4. **Irish Hospice Foundation:**

The Irish Hospice Foundation offers bereavement support services, including counselling, support groups, and information resources for individuals and families coping with loss.

The Grief Journey Ireland initiative provides practical guidance and compassionate support to bereaved individuals across Ireland.

5. **HSE National Office for Suicide Prevention (NOSP):**

The HSE National Office for Suicide Prevention coordinates suicide prevention and post intervention initiatives across Ireland, including support services for individuals affected by suicide loss.

The NOSP website offers information on grief support, self-care resources, and guidance for supporting others in grief.

Grief Support Services in the UK:

1. **Samaritans UK:**

Samaritans UK provides emotional support to individuals in distress, including those affected by suicide loss.

The helpline (116 123) operates 24/7, offering confidential listening, emotional support, and crisis intervention for individuals experiencing grief or emotional difficulties.

2. **Cruse Bereavement Care:**

   Cruse Bereavement Care is a UK charity offering support and counselling to individuals and families affected by bereavement, including suicide loss.

   Services include one-to-one counselling, support groups, and information resources tailored to specific needs.

3. **Mind UK:**

   Mind UK provides information and support for individuals affected by mental health challenges, including grief after suicide loss.

   Mind's website offers resources, helplines, and local support services to facilitate emotional well-being and access to appropriate support.

4. **Survivors of Bereavement by Suicide (SOBS):**

   SOBS is a UK charity dedicated to supporting individuals bereaved by suicide through specialized support groups, online forums, and information resources.

   SOBS offers peer support and a safe space for individuals to share experiences, find comfort, and receive practical guidance on navigating grief after suicide loss.

5. **Support After Suicide Partnership (SASP):**

   SASP is a network of organisations in the UK working collaboratively to improve support for individuals affected by suicide loss.

   The SASP website provides information on local support services, bereavement resources, and advocacy initiatives aimed at promoting awareness and destigmatisation.

Navigating Access to Services:

1. **Referrals and Self-Referral:**

   Individuals can access grief support services through referrals from healthcare professionals, community organisations, or self-referral directly to specialized support providers.

   Contact helplines, visit websites, or reach out to local mental health services for information on accessing grief support in Ireland and the UK.

2. **Community Outreach and Peer Support:**

   Engage with community-based initiatives, peer support networks, or local support groups to connect with others who have experienced similar losses and access compassionate support.

   Attend workshops, events, or commemorative gatherings that promote healing, resilience, and solidarity within the community.

Embracing Multidimensional Support:

1. **Counselling and Therapy Services:**

   Seek grief counselling, therapy, or specialized interventions from mental health professionals trained in trauma-informed approaches and suicide bereavement.

   Explore therapeutic modalities, such as cognitive-behavioural therapy (CBT), mindfulness-based interventions, or group therapy, to address grief-related distress.

2. **Peer-Led Initiatives and Advocacy Efforts:**

Engage in peer-led initiatives, advocacy campaigns, or grassroots movements aimed at raising awareness, promoting destigmatisation, and advocating for improved grief support services.

Contribute to community-based projects, storytelling platforms, or creative endeavours that foster empathy, understanding, and support for individuals affected by suicide loss.

By accessing grief support services and resources in Ireland and the UK, individuals affected by suicide loss can navigate their healing journey with compassion, resilience, and meaningful connections. Each person's grief experience is unique, and embracing supportive resources and community initiatives can promote emotional well-being and facilitate transformative growth after experiencing suicide loss.

In the subsequent chapters, we will continue to explore practical strategies, therapeutic interventions, and community initiatives aimed at supporting individuals and communities impacted by suicide loss.

9. Prevention Strategies and Early Intervention: Strategies for Suicide Prevention and Early Intervention

Suicide prevention and early intervention efforts play a critical role in reducing the incidence of suicide and providing timely support to individuals experiencing suicidal ideation or crisis. By implementing comprehensive strategies and fostering community collaboration, we can promote mental health awareness, destigmatise help-seeking behaviours, and save lives.

Understanding Suicide Risk Factors:

1. **Identifying Vulnerable Populations:**

   Recognise populations at higher risk of suicide, including individuals with mental health disorders, substance use issues, histories of trauma, chronic illness, or social isolation.

   Consider demographic factors such as age (e.g., youth and elderly), gender, socioeconomic status, and cultural influences that may impact suicide risk.

2. **Assessing Warning Signs and Red Flags:**

   Educate communities, caregivers, and frontline responders on common warning signs of suicide, including verbal cues (e.g., expressing hopelessness), behavioural changes (e.g., withdrawal), and situational triggers (e.g., loss or trauma).

   Encourage proactive screening and assessment of suicide risk in healthcare settings, schools, workplaces, and community organisations.

Comprehensive Suicide Prevention Strategies:

1. **Promoting Mental Health Awareness:**

    Launch public awareness campaigns to promote mental
    health literacy, destigmatise conversations about suicide,
    and raise awareness of available support services.

    Collaborate with media outlets, schools, workplaces, and
    community organisations to disseminate accurate
    information and encourage help-seeking behaviours.

2. **Enhancing Access to Mental Health Services:**

    Expand access to affordable and culturally competent
    mental health services, including counselling, therapy, crisis
    helplines, and peer support groups.

    Advocate for policy changes and funding initiatives that
    prioritise mental health resources and support suicide
    prevention efforts.

3. **Implementing School-Based Interventions:**

    Integrate suicide prevention education into school
    curricula, providing students, teachers, and parents with
    knowledge about risk factors, warning signs, and supportive
    resources.

    Establish peer support programs, mental health clubs, and
    crisis response protocols within educational settings.

4. **Training Frontline Responders:**

    Provide specialised training in suicide prevention and crisis
    intervention for healthcare professionals, educators, law
    enforcement personnel, and community leaders.

Equip frontline responders with skills in risk assessment, de-escalation techniques, and referrals to appropriate support services.

Early Intervention and Crisis Response:

1. **Establishing Crisis Helplines and Hotlines:**

   Develop 24/7 crisis helplines and hotlines staffed by trained counsellors and volunteers to provide immediate support and intervention to individuals in distress.

   Collaborate with emergency services and healthcare providers to ensure seamless referrals for individuals at risk of suicide.

2. **Implementing Gatekeeper Programs:**

   Train community members, caregivers, and trusted individuals (e.g., teachers, coaches, religious leaders) as gatekeepers who can identify and respond to individuals at risk of suicide.

   Empower gatekeepers to initiate conversations about mental health, provide emotional support, and connect individuals to appropriate resources.

Community Collaboration and Advocacy:

1. **Fostering Cross-Sector Partnerships:**

   Foster collaboration between government agencies, non-profit organisations, healthcare providers, schools, employers, and community stakeholders to develop holistic suicide prevention strategies.

   Coordinate efforts to address social determinants of health, promote resilience, and reduce systemic barriers to mental health care.

2. **Advocating for Policy Changes:**

Advocate for evidence-based policy changes that prioritise suicide prevention, improve access to mental health services, and allocate resources to address underlying risk factors.

Support legislation promoting mental health parity, crisis response protocols, and suicide prevention training mandates.

Promoting Resilience and Hope:

1. **Engaging Peer Support Networks:**

Encourage the establishment of peer support networks, survivor-led initiatives, and community resilience-building programs that foster solidarity and hope.

Amplify stories of resilience, recovery, and empowerment to inspire hope and reduce stigma associated with mental health challenges.

2. **Monitoring and Evaluation:**

Implement robust monitoring and evaluation systems to assess the impact of suicide prevention strategies, identify emerging trends, and inform continuous improvement efforts.

Utilize data-driven insights to tailor interventions, allocate resources effectively, and measure progress towards reducing suicide rates.

By implementing comprehensive suicide prevention strategies, fostering community collaboration, and prioritizing early intervention efforts, we can create a supportive environment that promotes mental health, reduces stigma, and saves lives.

Together, we can work towards a future where every individual has access to the support and resources needed to thrive.

In the subsequent chapters, we will continue to explore practical strategies, community initiatives, and advocacy efforts aimed at supporting individuals and communities impacted by suicide.

Reducing Suicide Risk through Community Outreach and Mental Health Education

Community outreach and mental health education play pivotal roles in reducing suicide risk by fostering awareness, promoting help-seeking behaviours, and building supportive networks within communities. By empowering individuals with knowledge, skills, and resources, we can create environments that prioritise mental health and prevent suicide.

1. Raising Awareness and Destigmatising Mental Health:

Public Campaigns and Events:

Launch public awareness campaigns, seminars, and community events to educate the public about suicide risk factors, warning signs, and available support services.

Collaborate with local organisations, schools, workplaces, and media outlets to amplify messaging and reduce stigma associated with mental health challenges.

School-Based Initiatives:

Integrate mental health education into school curricula, providing students with age-appropriate knowledge about emotional well-being, coping skills, and suicide prevention.

Empower teachers and school staff to identify signs of distress and connect students to supportive resources.

2. Promoting Help-Seeking Behaviours:

Crisis Helplines and Hotlines:

Promote awareness of crisis helplines and hotlines, ensuring that individuals in distress have access to immediate support and intervention.

Encourage community members to save crisis helpline numbers in their contacts and share them widely.

Gatekeeper Training:

Train community members, educators, healthcare providers, and frontline responders as gatekeepers who can recognise signs of distress, initiate conversations about mental health, and facilitate referrals to appropriate services.

Empower gatekeepers to create safe spaces for open dialogue and destigmatise help-seeking behaviours.

3. Building Supportive Networks and Resources:

Peer Support Programs:

Establish peer support networks, support groups, and online forums where individuals affected by suicide risk can connect, share experiences, and provide mutual support.

Encourage peer-led initiatives that promote resilience, empathy, and solidarity within communities.

Community-Based Services:

Expand access to community-based mental health services, counselling centres, and support groups that cater to individuals at risk of suicide.

Collaborate with faith-based organisations, cultural centres, and community centres to provide inclusive and culturally sensitive support.

4. Mental Health First Aid and Training:

Mental Health Literacy Programs:

Implement mental health literacy programs that equip community members with basic knowledge about mental health disorders, suicide prevention strategies, and crisis intervention techniques.

Offer workshops, trainings, and certification courses in Mental Health First Aid to empower individuals to respond effectively to mental health crises.

5. Engaging Vulnerable Populations:

Targeted Outreach Efforts:

Conduct targeted outreach efforts to engage vulnerable populations, including youth, elderly individuals, LGBTQ+ communities, and individuals with chronic illnesses or disabilities.

Tailor educational materials and support services to address unique needs, cultural considerations, and barriers to accessing mental health care.

6. Collaborative Partnerships and Advocacy:

Interagency Collaboration:

Foster collaboration between government agencies, non-profit organisations, healthcare providers, schools, law enforcement, and community leaders to develop comprehensive suicide prevention strategies.

Advocate for policy changes, funding initiatives, and systemic reforms that prioritise mental health education, community outreach, and suicide prevention efforts.

7. Evaluating Impact and Sustaining Efforts:

Monitoring and Evaluation:

Establish monitoring and evaluation mechanisms to assess the impact of community outreach and mental health education initiatives on suicide prevention.

Utilise data-driven insights to measure progress, identify areas for improvement, and inform continuous efforts to reduce suicide risk.

By engaging in community outreach and prioritising mental health education, we can empower individuals, families, and communities to recognise suicide risk, intervene early, and access supportive resources. Together, we can create environments that promote resilience, reduce stigma, and save lives.

In the subsequent chapters, we will continue to explore practical strategies, advocacy efforts, and community-based interventions aimed at supporting individuals and communities impacted by suicide.

The Importance of Addressing Self-Harm as a Warning Sign for Suicide Risk

Self-harm behaviours, such as cutting, burning, or other forms of intentional self-injury, are significant indicators of distress and can serve as warning signs for underlying mental health challenges, including suicide risk. Understanding the link between self-harm and suicide risk is crucial for early intervention, prevention, and effective support for individuals in crisis.

1. Recognising Self-Harm as a Distress Signal:

Expression of Psychological Pain:

Self-harm often represents a coping mechanism for individuals experiencing overwhelming emotional distress, psychological pain, or inner turmoil.

It may serve as a way to release emotional tension, gain a sense of control, or communicate underlying feelings of despair, hopelessness, or helplessness.

Cry for Help:

Self-harm can be a non-verbal communication of distress, signalling an urgent need for support and intervention.

Individuals may engage in self-harm as a way to externalize internal suffering and convey the intensity of their emotional turmoil.

2. Understanding the Link between Self-Harm and Suicide Risk:

Risk Factor for Suicide:

Self-harm is recognised as a significant risk factor for suicide, indicating heightened vulnerability and distress.

Individuals who engage in self-harm are at increased risk of suicidal thoughts, behaviours, and completed suicide, especially if underlying mental health issues remain unaddressed.

Escalation of Risk:

Self-harm behaviours can escalate over time, leading to increased severity, frequency, or lethality.

Persistent self-harm, particularly when accompanied by suicidal ideation or intent, warrants immediate attention and intervention to prevent further escalation.

3. Early Intervention and Prevention Strategies:

Identifying Underlying Factors:

Addressing self-harm requires a comprehensive assessment of underlying factors, including mental health disorders (e.g., depression, anxiety), trauma history, interpersonal conflicts, or environmental stressors.

Identify triggers and stressors that contribute to self-harm behaviours to develop targeted interventions and support plans.

Risk Assessment and Safety Planning:

Conduct thorough risk assessments to evaluate suicide risk among individuals engaging in self-harm.

Develop safety plans that prioritise harm reduction, crisis management, and access to supportive resources (e.g., crisis helplines, mental health services).

4. Destigmatising Help-Seeking Behaviours:

Promoting Open Dialogue:

Foster open and non-judgmental conversations about self-harm within families, schools, workplaces, and communities.

Encourage individuals to seek professional help, share their experiences, and access supportive resources without fear of stigma or shame.

Empowering Support Networks:

Equip caregivers, friends, and peers with knowledge and skills to recognise warning signs of self-harm and respond effectively.

Provide education on how to offer compassionate support, facilitate access to mental health services, and encourage engagement in recovery-oriented activities.

5. Collaborative Care and Holistic Approaches:

Integrated Mental Health Care:

Collaborate with multidisciplinary teams, including mental health professionals, primary care providers, therapists, and social workers, to provide integrated care for individuals struggling with self-harm and suicide risk.

Implement evidence-based interventions, such as dialectical behaviour therapy (DBT), cognitive-behavioural therapy (CBT), or trauma-informed approaches, to address underlying issues and promote recovery.

Trauma-Informed Practices:

Adopt trauma-informed practices that prioritise safety, empowerment, and trust-building when working with individuals affected by self-harm and suicidal behaviours.

Recognise the impact of trauma on self-harm and suicide risk, offering trauma-focused therapies and interventions to address underlying trauma.

6. Building Resilience and Recovery:

Strengths-Based Approaches:

Emphasise strengths-based approaches that empower individuals to develop healthy coping skills, build resilience, and cultivate a sense of self-worth beyond self-harm behaviours.

Encourage engagement in meaningful activities, hobbies, and supportive relationships to promote recovery and well-being.

Addressing self-harm as a warning sign of suicide risk requires a compassionate, informed, and proactive approach to mental health care. By Recognising the complex interplay between self-harm and suicide risk, we can intervene early, promote help-seeking behaviours, and save lives.

In the subsequent chapters, we will continue to explore practical strategies, therapeutic interventions, and community-based initiatives aimed at supporting individuals and communities impacted by self-harm and suicide risk.

10. Addressing Stigma and Promoting Mental Health: Breaking down Stigma Associated with Suicide, Self-Harm, and Mental Illness

Stigma surrounding suicide, self-harm, and mental illness can create barriers to help-seeking behaviours, exacerbate feelings of shame and isolation, and hinder recovery efforts for individuals in distress. Addressing stigma is essential for promoting mental health awareness, fostering empathy, and creating supportive environments that prioritise compassion and understanding.

1. Understanding Stigma and Its Impact:

Social Stigma:

Social stigma refers to negative attitudes, stereotypes, and discriminatory behaviours directed towards individuals affected by mental health challenges, suicide, or self-harm.

Stigma may manifest as fear, prejudice, avoidance, or marginalization, leading to social exclusion and barriers to accessing supportive services.

Self-Stigma:

Self-stigma occurs when individuals internalize negative beliefs about mental health, blaming themselves for their struggles and feeling unworthy of support or understanding.

Self-stigma can undermine self-esteem, exacerbate emotional distress, and impede recovery efforts.

2. Challenging Myths and Misconceptions:

Education and Awareness Campaigns:

Launch educational campaigns and initiatives to challenge myths and misconceptions about suicide, self-harm, and mental illness.

Provide accurate information, share personal stories of recovery, and highlight the prevalence of mental health challenges to promote understanding and empathy.

Media Representation:

Advocate for responsible media representation of mental health issues, encouraging accurate portrayals of suicide, self-harm, and recovery journeys.

Collaborate with media outlets to promote sensitivity, avoid sensationalism, and prioritise messages of hope and resilience.

3. Promoting Open Dialogue and Compassionate Conversations:

Encouraging Disclosure and Sharing Experiences:

Foster open dialogue about mental health within families, schools, workplaces, and communities, encouraging individuals to share their experiences without fear of judgment.

Create safe spaces for honest conversations, allowing individuals affected by stigma to express their feelings, seek support, and access resources.

Promoting Compassionate Language:

Advocate for the use of non-stigmatizing language when discussing mental health, emphasizing person-first language and avoiding derogatory labels or stereotypes.

Promote empathy, compassion, and active listening in interactions with individuals affected by suicide, self-harm, or mental illness.

4. Empowering Advocacy and Peer Support:

Empowering Advocacy Initiatives:

Support advocacy efforts led by individuals with lived experience of mental health challenges, suicide, or self-harm.

Amplify voices of advocacy to influence policy changes, promote destigmatisation, and increase access to supportive services.

Building Peer Support Networks:

Establish peer support networks, online forums, and community-based initiatives that empower individuals to connect, share resources, and offer mutual support.

Promote solidarity, resilience, and empowerment within peer-led support communities.

5. Integrating Mental Health into Holistic Care:

Collaborative Care Approaches:

Advocate for integrated mental health care that addresses physical, emotional, and social aspects of well-being.

Collaborate with healthcare providers, social services, and community organisations to ensure holistic support for individuals affected by stigma and mental health challenges.

6. Cultivating Resilience and Promoting Recovery:

Strengths-Based Approaches:

Emphasise strengths-based approaches that celebrate resilience, recovery, and personal growth.

Highlight stories of hope, perseverance, and transformation to inspire individuals affected by stigma and mental health challenges.

Addressing stigma associated with suicide, self-harm, and mental illness requires collective efforts to challenge stereotypes, promote empathy, and create inclusive environments that prioritise mental health and well-being. By breaking down stigma, we can foster resilience, promote help-seeking behaviours, and build communities that embrace compassion and understanding.

In the subsequent chapters, we will continue to explore practical strategies, advocacy efforts, and community-based interventions aimed at promoting mental health, reducing stigma, and supporting individuals and communities affected by suicide and self-harm.

Advocating for Mental Health Awareness and De-stigmatisation Efforts

Advocacy for mental health awareness and de-stigmatisation is crucial in promoting understanding, compassion, and access to support for individuals affected by mental health challenges, including those related to suicide and self-harm. By amplifying voices, challenging misconceptions, and fostering inclusive communities, we can create positive change and prioritise mental health as a fundamental aspect of well-being.

1. Amplifying Voices and Sharing Stories:

Personal Narratives:

Encourage individuals with lived experience of mental health challenges, suicide, or self-harm to share their stories openly and authentically.

Highlight diverse perspectives and experiences to illustrate the complexity of mental health issues and combat stereotypes.

Advocacy Campaigns:

Launch advocacy campaigns that amplify the voices of individuals affected by mental health challenges, emphasising resilience, recovery, and empowerment.

Utilise social media, storytelling platforms, and community events to raise awareness and inspire collective action.

2. Promoting Education and Knowledge:

Community Workshops and Training:

Organise educational workshops, trainings, and seminars to increase awareness of mental health issues, suicide prevention strategies, and stigma reduction.

Collaborate with schools, workplaces, and community organisations to integrate mental health education into curricula and training programs.

Media Literacy:

Advocate for media literacy programs that empower individuals to critically engage with portrayals of mental health in media and popular culture.

Promote responsible reporting and representation of mental health issues to combat stigma and promote accurate understanding.

3. Fostering Inclusive Environments:

Creating Safe Spaces:

Establish inclusive and supportive environments within families, schools, workplaces, and communities where individuals feel safe to discuss mental health openly.

Implement anti-stigma policies, diversity training, and cultural competency initiatives to promote inclusivity and reduce discrimination.

Peer Support Networks:

Strengthen peer support networks and community-based initiatives that provide emotional support, resources, and advocacy for individuals affected by mental health challenges.

Foster solidarity, empathy, and mutual understanding within peer-led support communities.

4. Advocacy for Policy and Systemic Change:

Policy Reform:

Advocate for policy changes that prioritise mental health care, increase funding for prevention and treatment programs, and enhance access to supportive services.

Collaborate with policymakers, government agencies, and advocacy organisations to influence legislation and systemic reforms.

Reducing Barriers to Care:

Address systemic barriers to mental health care, including stigma, discrimination, and disparities in access to services based on socio-economic status, ethnicity, or geographic location.

Promote equitable and inclusive mental health policies that prioritise early intervention, prevention, and community-based support.

5. Collaborative Partnerships and Community Engagement:

Interdisciplinary Collaboration:

Foster collaboration between mental health professionals, researchers, educators, policymakers, and community leaders to develop holistic approaches to mental health promotion and stigma reduction.

Engage diverse stakeholders in collective efforts to raise awareness, advocate for change, and promote mental health as a public health priority.

6. Empowering Advocacy Initiatives:

Youth Engagement:

Empower youth-led advocacy initiatives that mobilise young people as agents of change in promoting mental health awareness and challenging stigma.

Provide platforms for youth activism, peer support, and leadership development within mental health advocacy movements.

Advocating for mental health awareness and de-stigmatisation efforts requires sustained commitment, collaboration, and collective action. By amplifying voices, promoting education, fostering inclusive environments, and advocating for policy change, we can create a society that values mental health, prioritises compassion, and supports individuals on their journey towards well-being.

In the subsequent chapters, we will continue to explore practical strategies, advocacy initiatives, and community-based interventions aimed at promoting mental health awareness, reducing stigma, and supporting individuals and communities affected by mental health challenges.

11. Hope and Resilience: Emphasizing Hope as a Guiding Force in Suicide Prevention and Healing

Hope is a powerful force that sustains individuals in times of despair, encourages resilience, and fosters recovery from mental health challenges, including thoughts of suicide and self-harm. By emphasising hope as a foundational element of suicide prevention and healing, we can inspire courage, instil optimism, and cultivate pathways towards renewed well-being.

1. The Role of Hope in Suicide Prevention:

Inspiring Purpose and Meaning:

Hope provides individuals with a sense of purpose and meaning, anchoring them during periods of emotional distress and adversity.

Cultivating hope encourages individuals to envision a future beyond their current struggles, motivating them to seek support and engage in life-affirming activities.

Strength in Adversity:

Hope empowers individuals to navigate challenges, setbacks, and crises with resilience and determination.

It fosters adaptive coping strategies, problem-solving skills, and the belief that recovery and transformation are possible.

2. Cultivating Hope in Healing Processes:

Therapeutic Approaches:

Incorporate hope-focused therapeutic interventions, such as narrative therapy, solution-focused therapy, and mindfulness-based practices, into treatment plans.

Encourage individuals to explore personal strengths, values, and aspirations as sources of hope and motivation.

Building Supportive Relationships:

Foster supportive relationships with caregivers, peers, and community members who can provide empathy, encouragement, and validation.

Create opportunities for meaningful connections and social engagement to nurture hope and combat feelings of isolation.

3. Strengthening Protective Factors:

Positive Psychology Principles:

Apply principles of positive psychology to enhance protective factors, promote well-being, and amplify hopefulness.

Encourage gratitude practices, optimism exercises, and acts of kindness to cultivate a positive mind set and bolster resilience.

Goal Setting and Achievement:

Collaborate with individuals to set achievable goals and milestones, celebrating progress and fostering a sense of accomplishment.

Encourage the pursuit of personal passions, interests, and aspirations to instil hope and motivation for the future.

4. Empowering Stories of Recovery:

Sharing Inspirational Narratives:

Highlight stories of hope, resilience, and recovery from individuals who have overcome suicidal thoughts or self-harm behaviours.

Provide platforms for individuals to share their journeys, offering inspiration, validation, and encouragement to others facing similar challenges.

5. Promoting Self-Efficacy and Empowerment:

Strengths-Based Approaches:

Adopt strengths-based approaches that focus on individual capabilities, resources, and agency.

Empower individuals to take proactive steps towards recovery, engage in self-care practices, and advocate for their own mental health needs.

6. Building a Culture of Hope:

Community Engagement and Advocacy:

Engage communities in collective efforts to promote mental health awareness, reduce stigma, and foster a culture of hope and resilience.

Advocate for systemic changes that prioritise mental health support, early intervention, and accessible resources for individuals in crisis.

7. Embracing the Journey of Healing:

Mindfulness and Acceptance:

Emphasise mindfulness and acceptance as integral components of the healing process, allowing individuals to cultivate inner peace and emotional stability.

Encourage self-compassion and non-judgmental awareness to navigate emotional challenges with grace and resilience.

Emphasising hope as a guiding force in suicide prevention and healing empowers individuals to envision a future filled with possibility, purpose, and renewed vitality. By fostering hope, resilience, and positive transformation, we can inspire meaningful change and support individuals on their journey towards well-being and recovery.

12. Conclusion: Promoting Mental Well-being and Preventing Suicide

In this book, we have embarked on a comprehensive exploration of suicide, self-harm, and the profound impact of mental health challenges on individuals and communities. Through education, advocacy, and compassionate support, we have look into essential strategies for promoting mental well-being, fostering resilience, and preventing suicide. As we conclude this journey, let us reflect on key insights and inspire continued actions to prioritise mental health and save lives.

1. Embracing Compassion and Understanding:

Throughout this book, we have emphasised the importance of compassion and understanding in addressing suicide and self-harm. By fostering empathy, breaking down stigma, and promoting open dialogue, we create spaces where individuals feel valued, supported, and empowered to seek help.

2. Recognising Warning Signs and Seeking Help:

We have explored the complex interplay of risk factors, warning signs, and contributing mental health factors associated with suicide and self-harm. It is essential to recognise early indicators of distress, offer non-judgmental support, and encourage timely intervention to prevent crises and promote recovery.

3. Cultivating Hope and Resilience:

Hope serves as a guiding force in suicide prevention and healing. By emphasising hope, resilience, and the transformative power of positive thinking, we empower individuals to envision brighter futures and embark on journeys of healing and recovery.

4. Promoting Mental Health Awareness and De-stigmatisation:

We have advocated for mental health awareness and de-stigmatisation efforts, challenging myths, and misconceptions surrounding suicide, self-harm, and mental illness. By amplifying voices, promoting education, and fostering inclusive environments, we create communities that prioritise mental well-being and support individuals in distress.

5. Encouraging Continued Conversations and Actions:

As we conclude this book, let us commit to continued conversations and actions to promote mental well-being and prevent suicide. Together, we can advocate for policy changes, expand access to mental health services, and build supportive networks that prioritise compassion and empathy.

6. Inspiring Collective Responsibility:

Preventing suicide is a collective responsibility that requires collaboration, advocacy, and solidarity. Let us inspire change by engaging in meaningful dialogue, supporting those in need, and advocating for systemic reforms that prioritise mental health as a fundamental aspect of well-being.

7. Conclusion: A Call to Action:

In closing, I urge each of you to carry forward the insights and lessons shared in this book. Let us embrace hope, foster resilience, and champion mental health awareness in our communities. By working together, we can create a future where every individual feels valued, supported, and empowered on their journey towards mental well-being.

Remember, the conversation does not end here—it continues with each conversation, each act of kindness, and each step towards creating a world where mental health is prioritised, stigma is eradicated, and lives are saved.

Thank you for joining this important journey. Together, let us advocate for hope, resilience, and healing.

Dear Reader,

As we come to the end of this journey together, I want to extend a heartfelt invitation to you. Your pursuit in wellbeing is not a solitary one, and I'm here to offer my ongoing support and guidance in any way I can.

If you have questions, seek advice, or simply want to share your thoughts and experiences, please know that I am just an email away.

I am deeply committed to assisting you on your path to well-being, and I would be honoured to be a part of your continued journey.

Whether you're looking for clarification on a topic from this book, seeking personalised guidance, or just need a listening ear, please don't hesitate to reach out. Your wellbeing matters, and I am here to help you navigate the challenges and celebrate the triumphs that lie ahead.

Here's how you can connect with me:

Email: sean@seanoconnorcoaching.com

Website: www.seanoconnorcoaching.com

Feel free to drop me a line at any time. I am dedicated to providing you with the support and resources you need to continue your quest on building resilience.

With warm regards and a deep commitment to your success,

Seán O'Connor

Websites and Online Resources:

1. **American Foundation for Suicide Prevention (AFSP):** Provides comprehensive resources on suicide prevention, education, and support for individuals and families. Website: afsp.org

2. **National Suicide Prevention Lifeline:** Offers crisis intervention, support, and resources for individuals in distress. Website: suicidepreventionlifeline.org

3. **The Jed Foundation:** Focuses on mental health promotion and suicide prevention among college students. Website: jedfoundation.org

4. **Mind:** UK-based mental health charity offering resources and support for individuals affected by mental health challenges. Website: mind.org.uk

5. **Self-Injury Outreach and Support (SiOS):** Provides information, resources, and support for individuals struggling with self-harm behaviours. Website: sioutreach.org

Documentaries and Films:

1. *The S Word* (Documentary)

2. *Boy Interrupted* (Documentary)

3. *It's Kind of a Funny Story* (Film)

4. *Silver Linings Playbook* (Film)

5. *A Girl Like Her* (Film)

Academic Journals and Articles:

1. Suicide and Life-Threatening Behaviour (Journal)

2. Journal of Affective Disorders (Journal)

3. The Lancet Psychiatry (Journal)

4. "The Relationship Between Self-Harm and Suicide in Adolescents: A Critical Review of the Literature" by Paul Moran (Article)

5. "Risk Factors for Self-Harm in Adults" by Keith Hawton et al. (Article)

Training and Workshops:

1. Mental Health First Aid (MHFA) Training: Offers courses to teach individuals how to identify, understand, and respond to signs of mental illnesses and crises.

2. Applied Suicide Intervention Skills Training (ASIST): Provides practical skills and strategies for intervening with individuals at risk of suicide.

These resources can serve as starting points for individuals seeking to learn more about suicide prevention, self-harm, and mental health awareness. It's important to approach these topics with empathy, curiosity, and a commitment to promoting well-being within ourselves and our communities.

Organisations and Websites:

1. **Pieta House (Ireland):** Provides support and counselling for individuals at risk of suicide or self-harm, as well as support for bereaved families. Website: pieta.ie

2. **Samaritans (UK and Ireland):** Offers confidential emotional support for anyone experiencing feelings of distress or despair, including those contemplating suicide. Website: samaritans.org

3. **Aware (Ireland):** Offers information and support for individuals affected by depression and related mental health conditions. Website: aware.ie

4. **Mental Health Ireland:** Provides education, support, and advocacy for mental health in Ireland. Website: mentalhealthireland.ie

5. **Mind (UK):** National mental health charity in the UK providing information and support for individuals affected by mental health challenges. Website: mind.org.uk

Government and Health Service Resources:

1. **National Office for Suicide Prevention (NOSP) (Ireland):** Coordinates suicide prevention efforts and provides resources for individuals, communities, and professionals. Website: hse.ie/eng/services/list/4/mental-health-services/nosp

2. **NHS Mental Health Services (UK):** Provides information and access to mental health services and support available through the National Health Service. Website: nhs.uk/using-the-nhs/nhs-services/mental-health-services

Publications and Research:

1. **Health Research Board (HRB) (Ireland):** Conducts and funds research on mental health, including reports and publications related to suicide prevention and self-harm. Website: hrb.ie

2. **Office for National Statistics (ONS) (UK):** Provides statistical data and reports on suicide rates and trends in the UK. Website: ons.gov.uk/peoplepopulationandcommunity/birthsdeat hsandmarriages/deaths

Training and Workshops:

1. **ASIST (Applied Suicide Intervention Skills Training):** Offered in both Ireland and the UK, ASIST provides practical skills and strategies for intervening with individuals at risk of suicide. Website: livingworks.net/asist

2. **SafeTALK:** A suicide alertness training program that prepares participants to identify and support individuals with thoughts of suicide. Website: livingworks.net/safetalk

Helplines and Crisis Support:

1. **Samaritans (UK and Ireland):** Provides a 24/7 helpline for emotional support and crisis intervention. Phone: 116 123 (UK and Ireland)

2. **Pieta House (Ireland):** Offers a 24/7 helpline and crisis intervention services for individuals at risk of suicide or self-harm. Phone: 1800 247 247 (Ireland)

These resources are specifically focused on supporting individuals in Ireland and the UK who are affected by suicide, self-harm, and mental health challenges. They offer a range of services, from crisis intervention to long-term support and education, aimed at promoting mental well-being and preventing suicide within these communities.

Books from Ireland:

1. *Life After Loss: A Practical Guide to Renewing Your Life after Experiencing Major Loss* by Rita Milios

   - This book offers practical guidance and support for individuals navigating bereavement, including after the loss of a loved one to suicide.

2. *When Your Adult Child Dies: A Guide for Parents* by Jeanne Webster Blank

   - Specifically geared towards parents who have lost adult children, including those who have died by suicide.

3. *The Little Book of Sound by Self-Care* by Róisín Fitzpatrick

   - This book focuses on practical strategies and self-care techniques for managing stress, anxiety, and emotional challenges.

Books from the UK:

1. *Lost Connections: Uncovering the Real Causes of Depression – and the Unexpected Solutions* by Johann Hari

   - Investigates the underlying causes of depression and explores alternative approaches to mental health treatment and well-being.

2. *The Heartland: Finding and Losing Schizophrenia* by Nathan Filer

    - A personal account of the author's experiences working in mental health and his own journey with schizophrenia, providing insights into mental illness and recovery.

3. *The Recovery Letters: Addressed to People Experiencing Depression* edited by James Withey and Olivia Sagan

    - A collection of letters written by people who have experienced depression, offering hope, encouragement, and insights into recovery.

Books from Both Regions:

1. *Grief Works: Stories of Life, Death, and Surviving* by Julia Samuel

    - Explores the process of grieving and offers insights into how individuals can navigate loss and bereavement.

2. *Reasons to Stay Alive* by Matt Haig

    - A deeply personal memoir that discusses the author's struggles with depression and suicidal thoughts, offering hope and encouragement to others experiencing similar challenges.

3. *The Silent Scream: An Anthology of Despair, Struggle and Hope* edited by Emily Reynolds

    - A collection of essays, poems, and personal stories about mental health and recovery, aiming to break the silence around mental illness and promote understanding.